Dr. Keough's book is a one-stop shop for overall health with life changing methodologies. Using her strategies, I lost 60 pounds in 8 months without exercising, and my body is now in remission from autoimmune disease. Buy it! Use it! Enjoy life!

– Brigitte Ranae, Author and Life Coach

Dr. Felicity Keough-Bligh has made it possible for the general public to go beyond the media and allopathic care to take matters of health in their own hands. She provides an understanding and awareness of lifelong health and helps to open a new door to consumers who are seeking ways to enhance their health naturally. I recommend this engaging book which challenges us to reconsider some of our beliefs in clinical medicine. This is a wonderful contribution to our growing holistic health literature.

–Jayme Hanna, Holistic Esthetician and Owner of Birch Botanical Spa

Why can't all informational books be written like this? Concise, to the point, with just a touch of humor! I must say the author knows what she is doing! Didn't want to put it down. The doctor writes with confidence of her knowledge. From what I know, she is a novice writer, yet all I can say is, "keep 'em coming, Dr Keough! I look forward to more from you!"

– Ruth Hartstein, an avid reader

A book with enormous information on its subject. It taught me things I had no knowledge of. A thoroughly enjoyable experience. You don't have to be a certain age or sex to find its subject matter enjoyable and be a fantastic read. I was actually able to chime in on a conversation of which I was originally no part of, because of what I learned from Dr Keough's book! Thank you so much for this wonderful book, Dr Keough... I look forward to more!

– Allan Pearl, 30 plus years a pharmacist.

Dr. Keough brings to life what it is to struggle, learn, and overcome some of the many illnesses impacting our society. Her vulnerability opens up an understanding of hope for overcoming. Her book is truly a testimony of what it means to heal from within.

– Sefton Hale, Certified Personal Trainer and Mindset Coach

Dr. Keough-Bligh has my utmost admiration and respect due to her compassion and care in the health field. Reading this book has helped me gained an exorbitant amount of knowledge about our own bodies and what they are capable of doing, if given the chance. I appreciate the opportunity to read this amazing book and learn so much from it. This book is an absolute must!

– Tess Willer, Avid Health Conscience Enthusiast

Healing From Within

A SIMPLE GUIDE TO
LIFELONG WELLNESS

DR. FELICITY KEOUGH-BLIGH

HEALING FROM WITHIN

A SIMPLE GUIDE TO LIFELONG WELLNESS

For additional information on chiropractic services, nutritional advice, or functional medicine; or to discuss booking Dr. Felicity Keough for speaking engagements for your group or organization, feel free to email info@keoughchiropractic.com or visit her website at www.keoughchiropractic.com. Her new book, *Health & Harmony: Preconception, Pregnancy and Parenting,* will be available this spring.

HEALING FROM WITHIN

A Simple Guide to Lifelong Wellness

Dr. Felicity Keough-Bligh

ISBN- 978-1-7341840-0-6 (paperback)
978-1-7341840-1-3 (ebook)

TABLE OF CONTENTS

JOURNEY FROM SICKNESS TO HEALTH

My passion for health started when I was very young and was nurtured growing up as part of a health-conscious family. As I got older, I wanted to know as much about health as possible. I wanted to teach people. I wanted to be the expert in my community whom people could trust and come to for honest information about health. It's interesting to me that people in health and healing professions are typically drawn to their professions because of a need they have in their own lives. I've witnessed this in my own life as well as in the lives of many people I've met over the years.

I've always appeared to be a robust, healthy person on the outside, even as a child. However, as I got older, I experienced a host of health issues that drove me to dig deeper and find answers for myself. I believe in my heart that I was blessed with these health conditions, and that they led me to be the health care provider I am today.

I grew up in a chiropractic family and received my first adjustment when I was just a few days old. My paternal grandparents were chiropractors (class of 1947 and 1948) and the third chiropractors to open a chiropractic office in my hometown of St. Charles, Missouri. Having experienced chiropractic care at such a young age and seeing my family use it as the first line of treatment and primary mode of health care any time my sisters and I were ill, had allergy flares, or an injury (or just about anything else you can think of), I unfortunately took chiropractic care for granted. I stopped appreciating it.

My parents raised us in a very natural way. All of my sisters and I (I'm the oldest of four daughters) were born at home with a midwife and an family practitioner and doctor of osteopathic medicine. Dr. Fred Duhart (more commonly known as the Angel Doc), who served the St. Louis community for decades. He believed that women had a choice in how they wanted to give birth to their babies and was a powerful advocate for natural home birth.

My mother stayed home to care for us while my father worked two jobs, and they both ran a home-based business from the basement to help make ends meet. We ate healthy, homemade food every day, and my parents never let me buy my lunch at school, fearing I would eat "junk." I wouldn't have said we were poor, but we didn't have the money for new clothes or shoes too often. We sacrificed so much so my parents could put healthy food on the table and provide us with high-quality vitamin and mineral supplementation.

My parents didn't believe in vaccines, and I remember my sisters and I all had chicken pox and measles. My mother sought out "chicken-pox parties" so we could all contract the virus at the same time (something virtually unheard of today). In addition, one of my sisters had whooping cough, and another had scarlet fever. We all survived, and the interesting part of it all is I don't remember any of the dreaded childhood diseases threatening our lives. I'm fortunate now to have lifelong, natural immunity to these viruses that get so much hype today. Moreover, I never saw the inside of a hospital until I was twelve, when my dear maternal grandmother was dying of cancer. Don't get me wrong—my parents knew the value of Western medicine, but unless it was an emergency, we didn't use it.

When I was young, I didn't understand how these lifestyle factors would affect me later in life, but now I have a great appreciation for it all. My life started off with a great appreciation for and foundation of good health, as well as an understanding that health is something that comes from within us, not something we attain through pills, potions, or something outside us. We are all born with the innate wish to be healthy. My passion for creating a healthy life began with this foundational belief.

As I begin to unravel my tips for truly healthy living, I will explain some of my inner turmoil (mental and physical) that drew me to my current profession and the ways in which I chose to live my life now.

I'd like to go back to one of my earliest memories—my first day of kindergarten. Everyone remembers that day. For some, it's a day of happiness and joy. For others, it's a mix of positive and negative emotions; and for still others, it's a day of sadness, depression, and anxiety because you start your first day of school in a new environment away from your comfort zone. For me, it was the latter. I was sick over the thought of being in a new environment, away from what I'd known as my everyday life. I remember these days so vividly.

Today, having young children myself, I truly believe that it's all in how the parent prepares their young ones for this special day (or any big event, for that matter). I can't remember how my parents prepared me for this day, but my guess is it wasn't in the most positive way. Of course this wasn't intentional but perhaps how they themselves were raised? From that day forward, every time I walked into school and for the first several hours, my teeth would chatter, my shoulders would tense, and my stomach would be tied up in knots. After the first half of the day, those reactions would ease, and I'd feel somewhat better as the day progressed. I never thought much of it, and I never told anyone. Today I believe this is one of the underlying, contributing factors to my high anxiety and to some of the health conditions I dealt with later in life.

These feelings stayed with me until my junior year in high school, and I still never thought too much about it and never told anyone, including family. For reasons unknown, I endured this anxiety almost daily for nearly 14 years because it happened anytime school was in session.

Looking back, I believe I was afraid. From day one, I was afraid I would fail or make a mistake, and this fear of failure included a laundry list of items too long for this book. I was afraid that I would do SOMETHING wrong. At such a young age I was hyperaware of the possible situations that could result in someone not liking me or in my flunking a test, and the list goes on. Today I can laugh at that list. In fact, I did laugh for a long time until I realized it was the pattern that was running my life.

Years later, after undergoing hundreds of hours of counseling and talk therapy, I realized that the statement playing in the background of my life was, "Don't let anything go wrong."

We all have a statement or pattern humming in the background of our present lives. For me, it started here, in early childhood, and carried on up through high school and college. It even still shows up time to time in my currently life today: "I'm not enough."

I had anxiety about being out of my comfort zone and making mistakes. I always felt the need to prove myself for reasons that I'm still not sure I understand. I'm not even sure they were valid reasons. I internalized this stress, which contributed to health conditions that I would face later.

HEALTH PROBLEMS EMERGE

In addition to this negative internal talk, I also have early memories of my father telling me that if I didn't curb my large appetite, I would be "as big as a house" someday, and I remember kids calling me names such as "man" and "dude" when I was a young child in grade school and then when I was older in high school. I later found out it was because of my large muscles in my legs. This hurt me deeply because I felt as though something was wrong with my body. Why did my legs have to be so muscular? Why couldn't I have skinny legs like all the other girls? I was so afraid of being overweight.

These words from my father and kids at school stayed with me for some time before any eating-disorder patterns developed. As a kid, I was a voracious eater, always hungry, and I had high muscle tone and was always burning off tons of calories with my high activity and metabolism. As I approached my teens, I remember hearing that I "shouldn't" be eating so much anymore, that my metabolism would soon slow down and I could become overweight. My father meant well, and I'm positive he was simply trying to teach me that our metabolic rate slows down as we age. However, the impression it made on my young, fragile mind was "you're going be fat someday if you keep eating as much as you do."

THE PERFECT STORM

As I transitioned from eighth grade to high school, I had good friends and good grades, and I was lucky enough to be on the varsity cross country team. Then I started my period. If I could describe my period in one word, it would be "debilitating." My pain was so severe that it would double me over, and I would miss days of school each month, spending them at home with a heating pad on my abdomen and taking way too many Ibuprofens. This went on for years. Eventually, my grades slipped, I was pulled from varsity cross country, and my parents noticed I was no longer myself. I was becoming withdrawn and antisocial, which wasn't me. I remember feeling embarrassed because of all the school I was missing, and I couldn't understand why this was happening.

My eating disorder began around the same time as my period. When I was 15 years old, I made myself vomit for the first time. For many years after this incident, I alternated between bulimia and anorexia. I also developed irritable bowel syndrome (IBS) around this same time, and doctors and friends agreed that there was no cure for it; I was just going to have it for the rest of my life. (Apparently, IBS is very common, and everyone just deals with it.) I was never given a solution to help heal my IBS, which confused me because I knew from my upbringing that the body was made to heal itself.

I started my own research on healing the gut and tried many different remedies without the help of a trained physician. I tried numerous foods, pills, supplements, powders, potions, laxatives, enemas, and fasting—all of which made me worse. I believe these severe digestive problems and my IBS also contributed to my worsening eating disorder. The only time I felt like a normal human being was when I skipped a meal or fasted. One time, I fasted for three days because I felt so much better when I did. You can imagine how thin I was, eating only a few days each week. This frightened my parents, and they urged me to start eating more.

Eating was difficult though, as it made me so uncomfortable. I can remember needing to unbutton my pants at school each day after lunch. I can also remember clearing out a room after eating any food. It didn't matter if it was an apple or a salad. EVERYTHING made me bloated and gave me terrible gas and pain. Each day was humiliating and embarrassing. I would plan my outings with friends around how I was feeling or how long I could go without eating before hanging out for an evening with my friends. Planning my days consumed my life. Trying to fit in and feel like a normal person was so defeating.

Soon it was time to get a part-time job. Afraid that I would end up missing too much work because of my painful periods, I did what most young girls did and went on birth control for dysmenorrhea (painful periods). My parents did not advocate for medicating health problems, and I personally didn't believe in taking medications like birth control (because of my holistic upbringing), but I knew I had to do something. I had heard that birth control worked to help balance out hormones, and it was being prescribed for all my friends too. How bad could it be?

One day, I went to Planned Parenthood behind my parents' backs and learned from the nurses at the clinic that the Pill could help my period pain, clear up my skin, and potentially make my breasts larger. This all sounded amazing to me. However, after doing my research, I learned that the Pill had its downfalls too. It could also *cause* acne, make me moody and irritable, cause weight gain, and put me at higher risk for stroke and heart attack. I was conflicted!

My periods were so bad, but the thought of putting on weight literally made me sick to my stomach (yes, the weight gain scared me more than having a stroke or heart attack). Weight gain was one of those things that I could not and would not allow to happen to me under any circumstance because putting on weight meant shame and disappointment to my parents. If I was going to go on the Pill, I would have to find a way NOT to gain a single pound. Therefore, my bulimia and anorexia worsened.

During this war that was going on in my body and mind, I noticed something that seemed very positive. After being on birth control for one month, my cycle began, and I noticed I had no symptoms! Normally, I would feel my body gearing up for the misery that was soon to unfold. Premenstrual syndrome symptoms, cramping, nausea, and headaches were the normal precursors to the week from hell. But to my surprise, I started my cycle with NO SYMPTOMS! No pain, no missed school, no pain medications. I was able to participate in sports, and life continued like normal. I was so relieved the birth control worked!

This pattern kept up for a few months of being on the Pill, but then I noticed something disturbing. I felt some pain in the morning of the day I was to start my period, but I decided to tough it out and go to school. By lunch my mother had picked me up and taken me home, and I was downing Ibuprofen, trying get some relief. I hoped and prayed this cycle was a fluke and that things would get better next month. Well, things got worse. I felt tremendous pain the next month and was back to missing school with little to no help from pain medications. Eventually, everything was back to how it began, and I was depressed, discouraged, and feeling hopeless.

I decided there was no point in taking birth control if it was no longer working, so I stopped. I didn't consult a professional. I just threw away my prescription. What happened next was ironic because, from that point on, I did not have a cycle for almost five years. Deep down, I knew that because of my eating disorder, stress, and all the medications I had taken, my body hated me and had put me into a type of early menopause.

I went from doctor to doctor, hoping to find out what was wrong with me, only to be put on a list of medications (progesterone, clomid, different hormone creams)—all of which made me moody, irritable, and feeling awful. Nothing was working.

I also wasn't giving those doctors the full truth. I didn't tell them that I was struggling with an eating disorder. Had they known, they would have referred me to someone who could have helped me, but out of fear and stubbornness, I chose not to talk about it. I was finally referred to a different specialist who told me the next steps would be more invasive: they would need to go in and look around. It was frightening to discuss the possibility of surgery.

About this time, I was in college getting my degree in human biology. I developed a passion for understanding how the body worked and why birth control pills had affected my body so severely. One afternoon, while studying on campus, a friend told me to see her chiropractor who had helped with her hormone imbalance as well as her headaches. This sounded crazy to me—I was familiar with chiropractors and had never heard of them helping with hormones. However, I was not at all excited to have the exploratory surgery my last doctor recommended, so I decided to make an appointment with her chiropractor.

This chiropractor did a lengthy consultation and examination, took an in-depth history and X-rays, and asked for a food journal. Additionally, he ran lab work to check my body's blood chemistry and hormonal balance. He presented his findings to me in a follow-up visit and reviewed all the information he gathered in our initial visit. I was very impressed.

He took the time to explain my X-ray findings and the misalignments that were affecting my endocrine (hormonal) system as well as my gastrointestinal (digestive) system. I had never had back pain in my life, so I was surprised to see spinal misalignments. Next, he explained that my lab results revealed that my eating was not well-rounded and that it was important to eat greater quantities of whole, healthy foods, especially high-quality foods such as healthy fat and protein.

At this point, there were about seven foods I could eat without causing extreme digestive issues and upset stomach. If I strayed from those seven foods, my digestion would go into a tailspin, triggering my eating disorder. I was so hopeful when I learned chiropractic could aid my digestion by removing interference with the nerves that innervate my colon.

He explained that what I was experiencing had taken years to develop and that it would take time to get back to functioning normally, so he suggested I commit to a year of care. This was daunting and alarming because I was a college student with a part-time job and no health insurance. I was very skeptical, but he not only worked with me and made the care affordable, he also worked with my busy school and work schedules. I committed to a year, visiting him every week in the beginning and then less as the months went on.

As I started to receive care, I noticed with each passing visit that I felt better and better. Like I said, I had no back or neck pain, but I also didn't feel that good. For years, I had neglected getting regular chiropractic care for one reason or another, and I didn't realize how this made me feel over time. Once I committed to care and to a lifestyle change, within a few short weeks I noticed so many things improving: more energy, plus better mobility, sleep, focus, mental clarity, *and* digestion!

Thanks to him, I was able to make some drastic changes in my health that made a lasting impression on me.

In addition to my overall health improving, around the tenth month of routine chiropractic care and lifestyle change, I started my period again! For the first time in almost five years I had a period. I never thought I would be so ecstatic to start my period. What's more, I no longer needed Ibuprofen, and I was able to perform all my daily activities during my period instead of putting my life on hold like I had for many years prior.

This was a pivotal point in my life. As I added regular chiropractic care back into my life and made drastic lifestyle improvements, my path began to shift, and I became interested in the healing arts. I wanted to become a chiropractor just like my grandparents and the chiropractor that I was now seeing regularly. I began to realize that I had a love for understanding how the body works and helping people understand their own bodies. I shifted my college classes to pre-chiropractic and started as quickly as I could. I felt so good knowing what I wanted to do with the rest of my life. I wasted no time getting everything in order so that I could start on my path and begin changing lives—just like mine had been changed.

As a rule, people seek chiropractic care for pain management and rarely for support with body *function.* Additionally, most think it's unnecessary to see a chiropractor for long periods of time, especially if you're not in pain. However, pain is a terrible indicator as to whether you need chiropractic care or not. Approximately 11 percent of the population in our country see chiropractors, which shows how much work we must do to educate our patients and our community on the benefits of regular chiropractic care. Most of this small percentage use chiropractic for pain-based conditions, for which they receive outstanding results.

However, chiropractic was founded on a different philosophy, which my parents and grandparents understood very well: the brain and nervous system impact visceral-somatic function ("visceral" meaning "organs," and "somatic" meaning "body"). In short, if there is interference in the most important system, the nervous system, there may be dysfunction in the body. The people who saw my grandpa back in the 1950s, 60s, and 70s knew this well. Back then, people came in for pain relief because they worked on their farms for 10-plus hours per day, *but* they also used chiropractic for relief of cold and flu symptoms, digestive complaints, sleep issues, ear infections, and more.

It was much later in the century that chiropractic became mostly associated with pain, and as I grew up, I too lost sight of the fact that chiropractic helped me so much as a young child, mainly for non-pain (visceral-somatic issues) issues such as ear infections, viral infections, and allergies. I began using it only occasionally when I had an injury that caused some pain—much like the general society in which I was growing up.

My aha moment occurred when I overcame the health issues I was facing with my menstrual cycle, digestive system, and eating disorder. All through my teens, I had health issues that were causing me to suffer but which were not "bad" enough for me to seek help from the medical community. I began to heal and find a higher level of health after nearly one year of utilizing chiropractic care and changing my lifestyle. Chiropractic and living in accordance with good health became a way of life for me. It literally saved me, and I knew from that point on, I would strive to help others become aware of the benefits of chiropractic and healthy lifestyle.

In my humble opinion, chiropractic is the best, most humbling profession in the world. I feel so blessed to be able to do what I do each day, which means it does not ever feel like work to me. I think there's no better profession to help people heal from pain and disease naturally without the use of drugs or surgery.

PART ONE

WHAT IS HEALTH?

WHAT IS HEALTH?

Unless we are sick or in pain, we often do not think about or ask this question. In our culture, we believe that if we look good and feel good (or do not feel pain), we must be healthy. The problem with this is that we do not understand the true definition of "health," but if you look in any dictionary, you will find this definition of "health": "wholeness or optimal function." Plain and simple.

Notice that the definition does not mention the absence of pain or feeling good—or even looking good, for that matter. It is all about being a "whole, optimally functioning human being." My intention in writing this book is to help guide you through some of the hottest topics regarding health and wellness today, topics that my patients ask me about daily.

If you look at the numbers, as a nation we are very sick. Despite our "civilized," very clean ways of living, and despite our wealth (compared with Third World countries), we are one of the sickest nations in the world, even though somehow, we spend the most money on health care (currently somewhere around $2 trillion annually). According to the World Health

Organization, the United States is ranked thirty-seventh in the world when it comes to quality of health care.

In my opinion, the problem lies in the way we define health. From a very young age, we are taught that health is based on "feeling" not function. If we feel ill, we are sick. If we feel good, we must be healthy, and so we define health based on how we feel or look. As a result, we have an entire health care model based on this premise. So, if this is our premise, our objective is to remove the symptom (the pain or the problem). Now we're healthy, right? Wrong. You see, although symptoms can indicate a problem in our health, we have built an entire health care model around getting rid of symptoms instead of addressing why the symptoms are there in the first place.

Since we were children, we have been inundated with this false sense of what health is. Think about the millions of pharmaceutical advertisements telling us that when something isn't working in our life, it's because of a drug deficiency. The ads tell us we should talk to our doctor so that we can tell them what prescriptions we need. Think about all the food commercials telling us that pasteurized, homogenized, highly refined, and processed foods are "good" for us. (Okay, maybe they are not always saying it's good for us, but that is the underlying message.)

The three leading causes of death in our country are: cancer, cardiovascular disease, and autoimmune disease, with cardiovascular disease and autoimmune disease almost tied. Do any of those have symptoms? Usually not—at least not at the onset of the disease. Autoimmunity can be present decades before symptoms arise, and most of the time the first sign of a heart attack is death. We all have known or have a seen news story of someone who was fit and health-conscious who died of a heart attack or who was diagnosed with end-stage cancer and never felt ill at all. My point is that these leading causes of death do not usually have symptoms right away (if ever), yet symptoms are what we are taught to look for.

Wouldn't you agree that someone who died of a heart attack likely had some type of dysfunction in their body long before a heart attack occurred? What about the person who went to the dentist for an emergency visit because of throbbing pain in their mouth and was told they needed a root canal? Did they just develop a cavity overnight, or was the cavity silently (and painlessly) decaying more and more over the months until, finally, there was pain? What about the person who visited the chiropractor because of intense lower back pain? I have encountered this patient many, many times. Most of the time, the pain that developed was not due to some traumatic incident. Typically, there's been underlying spinal dysfunction happening for some time before pain manifests in the spine.

You see, *dysfunction* is not necessarily painful, and it does not necessarily cause symptoms. Long-term dysfunction is typically silent (unless you know what to look for), but it disrupts your optimal function and wholeness until, years later, pain and/or symptoms result.

WHERE DOES HEALTH COME FROM?

It's easy to get caught up in the latest health craze or fad, but if you want lifelong health, remember this: health—as defined by the general condition of the body or mind with reference to soundness and vigor—does not come from something outside us.

Despite what we are taught at a very young age, health does not come from a pill or a potion or even necessarily from eating the very best organic foods. Health comes from within us. When I ask people what the most important system in the body is, I hear "the heart," "the lungs," "the skin." While all those systems are VERY important and we could not live without them, they are not the most important. There is a system that controls all the body's organ functions, and without that system, our very important systems like the heart, lungs, and skin would not work. This system is the central nervous system. To remain healthy and continue functioning optimally, our nervous system must perform at its top level, which is exactly what chiropractic can do for you.

Several health topics will be explored in this book to help inform you as you consider your health choices. My approach to have great health is to keep up with regular chiropractic, consume only the best foods that are affordable for your family, drink purified water, remove as many toxins from your environment as possible, take control of your mind and what you allow yourself to focus upon, and surround yourself with like-minded individuals, as well as providers, who also understand what it means to be truly healthy. When you give your body what it needs, it will take care of you for a lifetime.

EXPRESSING HEALTH

One of my pet peeves is when people (especially chiropractors, for some reason) talk about how often they are NOT sick. It is totally normal to catch a bug every now and then, especially when we have young children. When we "catch" a cold or flu virus, our body is simply responding to a potential threat; therefore, when we become ill, it would be better to refer to it as an *expression of health.*

In our overly sterile environment, it is easy to fall into this trap. I did during our son's first year because no-one in the house was sleeping, and I was stressed, trying to learn how to care for a beautiful new baby. My poor body didn't stand a chance, so I was "sick" often.

We encounter so many bugs each day that have the potential to make us sick. Why do we sometimes get sick and sometimes remain healthy? It is dependent on the state of our immune system. Think about the trillions of cells we have inside and on our body, and then add a zero to that number to give you the number of bacteria we harbor. Next, add a zero to that number, and you will get the number of viruses we have within us at any one time. That is almost impossible to comprehend! So how does one little virus come in and make us sick? It is dependent on the state of the host at the time of contact with the virus. Give your body what it needs to remain healthy, and you will be healthy. However, "healthy" doesn't mean you will never "get sick."

I love the phase "expressing health," which simply means our body is doing what it is supposed to do when it comes in contact with a bacteria or virus. If our immune system can fight (depending on the state of our health at the time), we may or may not express symptoms. Symptoms such as fever, nausea, vomiting, diarrhea, rashes, mucous, sneezing, coughing, etc., are actually GOOD because they offer the body a means to excrete whatever pathogen needs to go.

When we take Imodium for our diarrhea or Mucinex for our mucous, is our body still as efficient in eliminating whatever needs to be eliminated? In my opinion, no. Think about food poisoning for a moment. If we eat something that has been tainted with harmful bacteria, shouldn't our entire body work as hard as it can to eliminate that food? What happens if we take medication to settle our stomach and help with the symptoms? The bacteria in the food is not properly eliminated, and unfortunately, it stays inside us, potentially causing harmful issues later. I understand that sometimes we just need some relief, but when we allow our body to have symptoms, we release what's necessary more efficiently. As a result, we can overcome our symptoms much quicker.

OUR PARTNERSHIP

So often, patients are unaware of the need to create a partnership when it comes to their health care. When I first went into private practice, I believed I could heal someone in one to five visits. If I could do that, I would be a great chiropractor. (I am not talking about maintenance. Trust me, I have always known the importance of spinal maintenance, which is something I practice routinely.) I believed that I could help restore function in just a handful of visits. While this might be possible for a tiny, new baby who has suffered a small amount of trauma and strain to the cervical spine and cranium during birth and who may need only a few adjustments to restore normal spinal and cranial function, most of us have been carrying around spinal dysfunction for years and years. If that is the case, let me assure you that one to five visits will not do the job. It will take time to heal.

TIME TO HEAL

Early on in your chiropractic care, you may begin to feel better, and that's a wonderful thing. However, it is important to remember pain is just a symptom that indicates there is a problem somewhere. You could be walking around completely pain free and still have dysfunction somewhere in your body. Our bodies are so resilient that we can harbor dysfunction for decades before the onset of pain. Pain is the last thing to show up and the first thing to leave once treatment begins, and thank goodness for that.

Multiple studies have shown that chronic pain has devastating effects on the brain. In most cases, the feeling of pain leaves rather quickly once correction to the dysfunction has begun, but that does not mean you are healed. Consider how you would feel if you broke your leg. Initially you would be in quite a lot of pain, but after weeks of being casted, the pain would dissipate. However, you would not take your cast off yet. Why? Because you know you are still healing and will remain in a healing state for the next several months.

This goes for orthodontics and exercise as well. With braces, teeth take years to shift where we want them, and after the braces come off, the retainer goes on. If braces could shift the teeth within a week or two, then taking off the braces too early would result in the teeth shifting back to their original alignment. With exercise and training, it takes time and work to get into the best shape of our life, whether we're training for a 5K, a marathon, a body-building competition, or the Olympics.

Lastly, think about childbirth for a moment. Women come home with the new baby and immediately start back into their routines. Even though we women may be feeling "okay" and may even have some of our energy back, it has been shown that postpartum women continue to heal for the entire first year of the baby's life. That is why ample time to relax and just be with the baby is so important. Unfortunately, for a variety of reasons, our culture doesn't make this easy. Most of us do not give our bodies time to heal and instead jump right back into work, exercise, and daily chores.

TAKING RESPONSIBILITY FOR OUR HEALTH

If you want vibrant health, you must take your health care into your own hands. No-one and nothing outside yourself can give you the health you have been seeking. We live in an advanced age of access to information and technology. We can Google any health question we desire. The problem with this is the source of information on the web. Are you getting the correct information or an answer that couldn't be further from the truth? With the abundance of information at our fingertips, it's difficult to know, however, that a commitment to learning what true health is will lead you there. Often this requires sorting through all the wrong information to find what is right.

When I went into private practice, my commitment was to be a lifelong learner of all things regarding health and to teach as many people as I could. This book is meant to guide you through some of those questions.

While researching and learning as much as we can regarding health and wellness, it is more important than ever before to consider how much time we spend in front of computers, laptops, cell phones, and tablets. These activities lead to a type of "micro-trauma" that affects our spinal structure every single day. Is it any wonder that back and neck pain are on the rise? In fact, according to the National Institute of Neurological Disorders and Stroke, low back pain in adults is the number one reason for disability and time missed from work. Children are also suffering from back and neck pain at incredibly young ages, due in part to all the electronic devices they access so frequently.

I learned very early on in chiropractic school that low back pain is very common in adults; in fact, it is the biggest reason the public seeks out chiropractic services. However, I was not aware that back pain in children is almost as common. My passion is treating children and pregnant women, so as I neared the end of chiropractic school, I developed a burning desire to help as many kids as I could (as well as adults) using chiropractic to restore *function*.

As stated earlier, chiropractic was founded on the principal of restoring function, not merely to help with pain control, which is, unfortunately, what most people think it is for. During my internship, I saw countless adults and children come in for help with colic, acid reflux, ear infections, constipation, sleep issues, night terrors, bed-wetting, high blood pressure, menstrual cramping, asthma, allergies, etc. I was eager to graduate and start my career so that I could help these people. Seeing patients with these types of issues would be so fun compared to providing boring pain relief all day. I was going to change the world, starting with our kids!

However, shortly after getting into practice, I learned that almost all patients seek our services for pain relief, for themselves AND their children. Even though I wanted to help everyone suffering from the list of former organ complaints and uncover the underlying dysfunction in the body that was creating these symptoms, I realized that most people became patients because they were in pain and that parents started their children with chiropractic care for pain, which I became very good at helping to alleviate.

In time, though, I realized that, during the course of their treatment, I could provide them valuable education on how the body works and begin teaching them why dysfunction in the nervous system could be contributing to other non-pain symptoms, which affect adults and children alike. Now, when people come to receive chiropractic for pain, I see that as an amazing blessing. Patients get the help they need AND they become educated on how the body really functions, which gives them an opportunity to take responsibility for their own health care.

BIRTH STATISTICS, TECHNOLOGY, VACCINES, AND OUR HEALTH

Considering the amount of money our country spends on health care, it is hard to believe that hundreds of women die each year from causes related to pregnancy or childbirth, but they do.

According to National Public Radio, black women have a maternal mortality rate three times higher than that of white women, and most of these maternal deaths are preventable. Many hospitals, including those with intensive care units for newborns, are often unprepared for a maternal emergency. Lastly, in the United States, some doctors entering the growing specialty of maternal-fetal medicine complete their training without ever spending time in a labor-delivery unit.

According to *The CIA World Factbook*, the total number of infant deaths is 5.7 out of 1,000 live births (6.2 deaths for males and 5.2 deaths for females).

Ultimately, a mother is more likely to die in childbirth than her baby, and most of those deaths are preventable. Every year, mothers continue to lose their lives due to complications from childbirth that we know how to prevent. Sadly, many other countries are doing it better than us.

The number of Cesarean births continues to rise in our country, from about 23 percent in 1990 to almost 33 percent in 2013, according to National Center for Health Statistics.

Fetal ultrasounds are so common today that it is not possible to find statistics on how many people use or do not use them. Clinical use of diagnostic ultrasound imaging during pregnancy has a long history of safety and diagnostic advantage, as supported by numerous human case reports and epidemiological studies. However, there exists in vivo studies linking large but clinically relevant doses of ultrasound applied to mouse fetuses in utero to altered learning, memory, and neuroanatomy of those mice. The results suggest that fetal exposure to diagnostic ultrasound applied in utero can alter typical social behaviors in young mice that may be relevant for autism.

Vaccine numbers have risen dramatically. In fact, in 1953 the CDC (Centers for Disease Control) recommended 16 doses of four vaccines (smallpox, DPT) between two months and six years of age. In 1983 the CDC recommended 23 doses of seven vaccines (DPT, MMR, polio) between two months and six years of age, and in 2013 the CDC recommended 50 doses of 14 vaccines between the day of birth and six years of age, as well as 69 doses of 16 vaccines between the day of birth and 18 years of age. Despite this vast increase in vaccinations, we cannot ignore the epidemic of other chronic disease and disability plaguing the children in our country—the most highly vaccinated children in the world and among the most chronically ill and disabled. Over the past five decades, the epidemic of chronic disease and disability among children has increased dramatically, despite the increase in recommended vaccines and other medical interventions.

Our nation, culture, and medical system are failing miserably when it comes to childbirth and children's health. The CDC, *The Journal of the American Medical Association*, and the National Cancer Institute report that one in 68 children are diagnosed with autism, one in thirteen have food allergies, one in 10 children have asthma, one in six have developmental disabilities, and cancer remains the leading cause of death by disease in children.

I am not here to argue whether birth interventions, labor induction, C-sections, vaccinations, multiple fetal ultrasounds, and other interventions and medical procedures are safe. I'm sure there are many parents reading this who have had these types of procedures and have perfectly healthy, happy, well-adjusted children. That is not my point. What I want to do is shed light on the fact that as a nation, we are among the worst at health care and have some of the sickest children, despite the trillions of dollars spent each year and the increasing number of medications and procedures recommended.

I don't understand all the unnecessary interventions that medical providers present as routine, many of which are not supported by data. If we really look at the data, we will see for ourselves things don't make sense. My hope is to inspire you to take your family's health into your own hands and to start researching some of the above-mentioned procedures. If you have simply trusted what the medical establishment says about any and every health topic, procedure, or prescription, I encourage you to begin researching your questions on your own, as well. I'm not telling you to stop listening to your doctor, but I am asking you to keep an open mind and do your own research.

Ask to see the inserts that come with the vaccinations so that you can see what ingredients are contained in them and what side effects are possible. Get second and third opinions from both traditional and holistic practitioners if you aren't sure about your medical diagnosis. If you are pregnant and want a low-intervention birth, seek a natural-minded obstetric doctor or midwife. The health of our children depends on us as parents to start asking different questions. I am positive we can change the tide and improve the health of our children and subsequently, that of our country.

RESPONSIBLE PARENTING

I understand it can be difficult to discuss responsible parenting because every parent wants the best for their child. I was fortunate to be raised in a family who had a firm understanding of chiropractic care and good nutrition, but as I grew older, I continually did things to damage my metabolism and destroy my health with food (by starving, binging, and purging) at very vulnerable points in my development. It's true, everyone's circumstances are different. Maybe you have a child who has started developing bad food habits. Maybe they only want to eat chicken fingers. Maybe they refuse to drink enough water. Whatever your circumstance is with your children, all these habits, if not corrected by the parents, will lead to damaging health effects later in life. If you could, wouldn't you want to avoid all that for your child?

I have worked with many overweight and obese children in my career, and unfortunately, the hardest part is their parents, which I say in the most loving way. Please, parents, read this with an open mind. Do not mistake youth for health. Children have something called massive cell turnover and a completely flexible, impressionable metabolic system, which is why so many adult health issues can stem from the developmental years. Do not fall into this same trap and mistake youth for health just because your child seems fine or seems to bounce back quickly.

In working with so many parents, one of the worst things I hear is that parents will make a healthy meal for themselves and a separate, completely different, unhealthy meal for their children. Why would we do this to our kids? Are we telling ourselves "my kids are picky," or "they are growing and need the calories," or "they are healthy and don't have my issues?"

In some cases, there are actual nervous system issues that children have that cause sensory disturbance and affect their ability to tolerate certain textures. Seeking out a trained pediatric chiropractor to improve their nervous system function and an occupational therapist to help with sensory integration may help.

Given our society's skewed definition of health and the importance we all place on convenience, I understand why a busy, overworked parent would adopt this mindset. However, when we know better, we do better, and, parents, this is completely unacceptable. Yes, kids are growing—they are growing their hormonal, digestive, neurological, cardiovascular, and mental systems right before our eyes. By the time they are 16 to 18 years old, some of those systems are set for life and will be weaker or stronger based on how they developed and what we (and our households) exposed them to.

When I first started in private practice, I found it difficult to speak up to parents when I heard something like, "But, Doc, my kids will only eat chicken fingers, cheese, and hot dogs." I was young and didn't understand yet what it was like to have children or how *hard* it was. Now, though, I have the desire to ask parents harder questions about their kids' "pickiness." Depending on the age of your child, it may be pertinent to ask yourself: *Does my child shop for food yet? Do they have a vehicle to drive to the store and purchase junk? Do they know how to cook yet?* For those of us parents with young children, most of these are a "no." As parents, we have the responsibility to buy it, cook it, prepare it, and serve it to them. They are growing up in our house and under our influence.

Our children *will* eat healthy food, but not if we have mountains of junk in our house. If we have health or weight issues, we must understand that whatever is driving those issues in us is driving them in our children too—whether we can see it or not, whether our kids can feel it or not—and it is happening at a faster rate than it is in adults. This is scary, but true.

Children often do not feel the symptoms that we adults do, nor do they easily express what they feel. When a child is overweight, though, that can tell us a great deal about their health. A child who is overweight has a stressed-out body. Their liver, kidneys, digestive tract, heart, and respiratory system are all stressed and working harder than they should. There are more oxidative stress and inflammation than necessary. Plus, their reaction to food—mainly to insulin—will influence the vulnerable mechanisms of their hormonal feedback loops, which will increase as they mature and continue developing.

As children hold onto or gain extra weight, high amounts of insulin are damaging their system, lowering human growth hormone (HGH), interfering with estrogen and testosterone, and priming cortisol for hyper-responsiveness, which we do not want to happen to our children. Insulin and high blood sugar not only cause the extra weight, but they also stress the developing brain, change their mood, create addictions, and influence their energy output.

I completely understand this may be difficult to read or that you may not be interested in taking this seriously for yourself, but please do it for your children. Get them involved and share with them your health concerns for you and your family. Build your team and create your tribe. There are so many people and resources out there to help and guide parents making this shift. The go-to habits your children learn now will be around for the rest of their lives, so make them amazing!

I want you to decide what it means for you to become truly healthy. My vision is that our country will raise its standards! Our bodies want to heal from within—if we would just give them the opportunity to do so. Heighten your awareness. Take your health and the health of your children into your own hands.

Here's to your happy, healthy future!

PART TWO

WHAT IS CHIROPRACTIC?

WHAT IS CHIROPRACTIC?

The word "chiropractic" comes from the Greek words *praktos* and *cheir*, which mean, together, treatment by hand.

As a health profession, chiropractic is concerned with the innate or inborn intelligence of the human body. Our brain and nervous system orchestrate this intelligence and, because of that, millions of vital bodily functions as well. Messages are sent from our nervous system to the cells and organs of our body, directing functions such as respiration, digestion, growth, and immune response. Our nervous system also directs our ability to think and concentrate, as well as our energy levels and quality of sleep.

Our innate intelligence operates so perfectly that most of us are completely unaware of it. Typically, we only become aware of it when our body is no longer able to adapt to the repetitive stressors—physical (traumas), chemical (toxins), and emotional (thoughts/feelings)—that we place upon it. At this point, our body and our health become compromised.

The chiropractic profession was founded by a man named D. D. Palmer in the United States in 1895 when he discovered that specific spinal adjustments could assist in the removal of nerve interference. A misalignment of one or more vertebrae is called a "vertebral subluxation complex" and results in altered joint movement and altered neurology. This irritation can affect communication between the brain and body and, when left unresolved, can alter the state of health and balance of the body. This can foster a decrease in health that results in sickness and disease.

The philosophy of chiropractic recognizes that the body has self-healing and self-regulating abilities that enhance health and well-being. By assessing the spine and other various indicators in the body, a chiropractor is trained to identify nerve irritation that affects these regulating systems. Once this nerve irritation is assessed and removed through chiropractic adjustment, the body can establish order and balance. Chiropractors are doctors of the nervous system and can work with core issues of health, rather than looking for signs and symptoms of pain and disease.

Millions of people of all ages benefit from chiropractic, which is one of the largest, drug-free, natural health care professions in the Western world. Chiropractic doctors focus on correcting vertebral subluxation and have an expertise in health through their knowledge of the spinal and nervous systems.

Vertebral subluxations have many causes and occur throughout our lifetime as we endure those same physical (trauma), chemical (toxins), or emotional (thoughts/feelings) stressors just mentioned. Subluxations especially occur when we are young and learning how to crawl, climb, creep, walk, and ride our bikes. Studies have shown that spinal misalignments can even be caused throughout gestation due to a mother's imbalanced and misaligned pelvis or the position of the baby within the womb.

This is a reminder that healing takes time. Early on in your chiropractic care, you may begin to feel better, and that's a wonderful thing. However, it is important to remember pain is just a symptom that indicates there is a problem somewhere. You could be walking around completely pain free for decades and still have dysfunction somewhere in your body that occurred when you were an infant or young child. Our bodies are so resilient that we can harbor dysfunction for decades before the onset of pain. Pain is the last thing to show up and the first thing to leave once chiropractic treatment begins—thank goodness.

Chiropractic is a definite science, art, and philosophy that boosts the body's natural function and inherent health. Chiropractic treatments, or adjustments to the spine and soft tissues that affect the nervous system, are anchored in solid, proven scientific principles with top health experts leading chiropractic research around the globe. Today, there are more than 70,000 active chiropractic licenses in the United States, and chiropractic is officially recognized as a health care profession in all 50 states, the District of Columbia, Puerto Rico, and the U.S. Virgin Islands. Many other countries also recognize and regulate chiropractic, including Canada, Mexico, Great Britain, Australia, Japan, and Switzerland. Chiropractic doctors assist in optimizing the health and function of your spine, therefore enhancing your well-being, and they can guide you and your family toward a healthy, proactive life.

WHO WAS D.D. PALMER?

A medical trailblazer and the father of modern chiropractic, D.D. Palmer remains, even a century after his death, an inspiration (or an eccentricity) to many practitioners of the field of medicine that he founded. A prolific reader of all things scientific, Palmer realized that although various forms of manipulation had been used for hundreds if not thousands of years, no-one had developed a philosophical or scientific rationale to explain their effects. Palmer's major contribution to the health field was therefore the codification of the philosophy, art, and science of chiropractic, which was based on his extensive study of anatomy and physiology.

Born in Ontario in 1845, Palmer was always fascinated with the medicinal practices of his day, such as magnetic healing, phrenology, and spiritualism (a widely accepted theory that science and mystic rituals such as séances could reveal the secrets of death and the afterlife, among other things).

When Palmer was 20, he moved to Iowa, making his living as a beekeeper, fruit merchant, grocer, and school-teacher. In September 1895, Palmer met Harvey Lillard, the building's janitor, who told Palmer that he had become deaf 17 years prior, after he felt something "give" in his neck. Palmer examined the area and gave an "adjustment" to what was felt to be a misplaced vertebra in his neck. The janitor then observed that his hearing improved.

Palmer theorized that the two maladies were connected and, as he claimed, cured Lillard of his deafness by making two adjustments to Lillard's displaced vertebra. He similarly cured another patient's heart disease utilizing this technique. Many consider this to be the beginning of chiropractic medicine.

A year later, Palmer founded the Palmer School of Magnetic Cure, later rechristened the Palmer School of Chiropractic. Following the first adjustment, many people became interested in Palmer's new science and healing art. Among his early students were Palmer's son, Bartlett Joshua (BJ), as well as members of the older healing arts of medicine and osteopathy. The first state law licensing chiropractors was passed in 1913, and by 1931, 39 states had given chiropractors legal recognition.

The medical discipline he pioneered has evolved over the years and now provides a variety of important health benefits to millions of people all over the world. In particular, today's chiropractic physicians are recognized as experts in diagnosing and treating conditions related to the musculoskeletal and nervous systems. They have also emerged as leading proponents of lifestyle changes, including improved diet and nutrition as well as exercise habits, that can prevent many chronic health problems.

THE PREMISE BEHIND CHIROPRACTIC

The basic premise of chiropractic philosophy is this: *The power that makes the body heals the body*. This vitalistic force is constantly at work in all living things, keeping them organized and adapting to the forces in their environment. This life force is the vibration that keeps all life moving forward and that holds every cell and particle together. The ordinary man is not usually aware of this vibrational frequency, nor is he always mindful that this force maintains his life as well as the Earth itself.

The human body is simply miraculous. This principle of organization produces a self-healing, self-organizing, self-regulating organism that is adapting and appropriately responding to its environment, constantly striving for optimal function. In chiropractic, this is known as "innate intelligence."

Healing can be a matter of time, but it can also be a matter of opportunity. Health is a state of balance and harmony of the body within the larger environment. The body wants to heal and be well, and it does so using its own recuperative power, keeping in mind that all body processes take time and that healing is a process. It is not the bandages that heal the paper cut, nor the cast that causes the bone to reunite. A bandage can be put on a cooked roast, but it will not heal itself because the roast is no longer a living thing and therefore has no innate intelligence. Only the living organism can heal itself.

Healing the body is a dynamic process, and with time, the changes take place. The path to health is not an easy process, especially in the beginning, because it takes time to change lifestyles and old habits. As the body begins healing, the changes will be very noticeable at times, and other times the changes will not be apparent. We must not be discouraged by this.

When we continue on our path toward a healthier lifestyle and establishing new habits, the body will undergo deep cellular healing at the appropriate time. When it does, most people comment that they are still in pain, they are plateaued with weight loss, or they are still dealing with certain symptoms. If this happens, we can't give up. The body is doing deep work behind the scenes when this happens. We need to be patient and continue our health journey. Ultimately, each small change will lead to the greatest changes of all—optimum health, full potential, and the ability to have a full, amazing life.

HOW IS CHIROPRACTIC DIFFERENT FROM OTHER FORMS OF HEALTH CARE?

Chiropractic health care has also grown beyond spinal manipulation to include other manual therapy, such as soft-tissue mobilization and massage, instrument-assisted soft-tissue mobilization, the McKenzie approach (which emphasizes patient empowerment to pain conditions of the spine and extremeites), to mechanical diagnosis and therapy; stabilization and strength-training exercise, nutrition and postural programs; and the incorporation of a cognitive-behavioral treatment regimens.

More importantly, a growing number of chiropractors are treating more children and pregnant women. In pregnancy, women are more likely to undergo subluxation of the pelvis due to the changes that occur in pregnancy, which makes chiropractic a natural, safe, effective option for all pregnant women, especially those dealing with hip pain, lower back pain, and sciatica. In addition, the birth process (whether all natural or very difficult) places a large amount of stress on an infant's cranium and cervical spine, stress that can be addressed only by a trained pediatric chiropractor. Some of the symptoms that occur when a baby has subluxation after birth are digestive disorders, colic, reflux, ear infections, poor immune function, sleeplessness, disliking tummy time, problems with latch and milk transfer, delayed milestones, etc. (For additional information, see my book *Health & Harmony: Preconception, Pregnancy and Parenting* and other resources on www.keoughchiropractic.com.)

Chiropractic offers countless benefits over other forms of health care. As we just mentioned, chiropractic can help address problems that are distant from the proximity of the spine. For example, that persistent, recurring pain in your extremities might actually be caused by an issue in the spine. Chiropractic care can be the solution to headaches, neck and back pain, stiffness, and other ongoing issues that impact organs that may have affected the person for years. Whether the cause is from poor posture, an injury, genetics, or other factors, chiropractic can help address the issues and relieve pain and discomfort by removing nervous system interference.

Keep in mind that when seeking care from a medical doctor for pain relief, you will most likely be prescribed pain medication, muscle relaxers, or anti-inflammatory drugs. These drugs only mask the issue; they do not address why you are having the pain. If you seek treatment from an orthopedic doctor, they may suggest surgery.

A chiropractor, however, will address and treat your spinal problems by hand, through manipulation of the spine, if that is what the assessment warrants. If you need medical attention or an orthopedic doctor, chiropractors have a good understanding of when to refer you to the appropriate provider. I recommend that chiropractic care always be the first treatment option before more invasive options like drugs and surgery are explored.

WHAT IS THE DIFFERENCE BETWEEN VITALISTIC AND MECHANISTIC APPROACHES TO HEALTH?

Recent years have seen an increased interest in "alternative health care," including holistic medicine, a system that focuses on areas such as personal accountability for one's health, the human body's ability to heal itself, and balancing the body/mind connection.

Chiropractic care is becoming more and more mainstream. In fact, chiropractic is the third largest doctoral-level primary health care profession, behind medicine and dentistry. Although there are over 100 different chiropractic techniques, doctors of chiropractic all fall into one of two general categories: mechanistic or vitalistic. In fact, you will find that most health care practitioners fall into one of these two categories.

Vitalism can be defined as the belief that we were created by God (or some other higher power), and that God makes us alive and coordinates all functions of life. That means that we are self-healing and self-regulating. We are born with an innate intelligence that sustains and nourishes every part of our body, including growth, cell function, healing, thinking, and the immune, digestive, respiratory, circulatory, and reproductive systems.

Vitalistic (wellness) chiropractors view the body as a whole. They see the body as innately intelligent, responding with a purpose to its environmental stressors. Symptoms are seen as an intelligent response to stress and are to be listened to and acknowledged, not suppressed or eliminated. Vitalistic care tends to be personalized to the unique needs of the individual. Vitalistic chiropractors are great for both short- and long-term results, as well as for getting to the root of the problem and for preventative care.

Mechanism is the opposite of vitalism because mechanism says that the body is the sum of its parts. Mechanism doesn't believe that those parts work intrinsically together. (In vitalism the body is much greater and more powerful than the sum of its parts.)

Mechanistic (pain-based) chiropractors view the body as a machine that is separated into different parts. Like any machine, the body's parts break down and can often be replaced or manipulated without regard to the whole. These chiropractors see symptoms as signs of breakdown that need to be removed or eliminated, and they tend to apply the same theory to all bodies, ignoring the individualism of each patient. Mechanistic chiropractors are great for a quick fix as they take away your pain quickly, but they do not help you to truly live the wellness lifestyle. Depending on their preference, this may be the perfect "quick" fix someone needs.

IS CHIROPRACTIC SAFE?

Chiropractic is very safe and natural. It is widely recognized as the largest drug-free health care profession in the world. Chiropractic is used to treat a variety of conditions, including headaches, neck pain, back pain, and numbness or pain in the extremities, just to name a few. Because chiropractors are well educated in the musculoskeletal and nervous systems, they are well suited for the management of these disorders.

Many patients feel immediate relief following their first chiropractic adjustment, while some may experience mild soreness or aching after the initial adjustment. With continuation of care and proper home care (such as ice and rest), however, this can be easily managed. This discomfort commonly happens because muscles are tight around the area being adjusted or because the patient tenses up during the adjustment. It is similar to the soreness you might experience after you exercise. Research shows that this soreness usually goes away within 24 hours.

In addition to being safe, chiropractic is extremely effective in treating several musculoskeletal conditions. For example, research has shown that chiropractic is very effective in helping with lower back pain. A study published in the *Journal of Manipulative and Physiological Therapeutics* demonstrated that chiropractic is more effective than medical care in treating chronic low back pain in patients who were experiencing the symptoms for one year or less.

Chiropractors also effectively help people suffering with neck pain, which is often caused by misaligned vertebrae in the neck or cervical spine. When these bones become misaligned, the joints can become stuck and irritate the nerves in the neck, which can also cause muscle spasms and further subluxation of the joint; this results in a vicious cycle of pain and symptoms. Chiropractors call this a subluxation, fixation, or a misaligned vertebrae, which are the terms I will use throughout this book. Once the subluxation is identified, chiropractors perform specific adjustments to correct the misaligned bones and restore proper motion to the joints. This helps to restore normal nerve flow to all areas of the body that correlate with that particular area of the nervous system. It also helps to relieve muscle spasms in the area as well. Chiropractic adjustments can be performed with specific hands-on adjustments or the use of instruments.

HOW DOES CHIROPRACTIC DEFINE WELLNESS?

Most of us associate chiropractic care with back and neck pain. After all, chiropractic care does an amazing job with conditions associated with the spine. However, chiropractic care is not limited to just one kind of condition or area of the body. In most sports, teams have their own in-house chiropractor to help players, athletes, and staff with their fitness and wellness concerns. But what about all the hype with "wellness chiropractic" and all that it claims to do? What's it all about, and should you consider a wellness chiropractor? If yes, how would you choose a clinic?

The premise of wellness chiropractic care is the focus on removing nerve interference to the central nervous system (CNS) so that your body can heal itself. The CNS controls primary functions of the body, and utilizing chiropractic care, it is possible to eliminate the interference that eventually impacts the CNS and that may cause pain and other health issues. Many factors lead to subluxation, but in most cases, lifestyle factors and the level of physical activity have a considerable influence. Wellness chiropractic is all about general wellness and living the life of your choice. You don't have to be sick or in pain to seek the expertise of a chiropractor.

A wellness chiropractor will improve the function of your spine, which will assist in restoring the natural energy levels of the body. They will minimize and remove the interference in the nervous system so that the body and mind are in sync with one another. By minimizing subluxations in the spine, your body will be at its best to heal. This process will impact the overall biochemical system as well.

IF CHIROPRACTIC IS SO GOOD, WHY DO SO FEW PEOPLE SEE CHIROPRACTORS?

According to various polls and questions asked of the public, more than 50 percent of the population indicate they would consider visiting a chiropractor. For the last 40 years, however, the percentage of people who actually do so has remained the same. While more people see chiropractors than ever before, consistently only 10 percent of the population does so.

In spite of the benefits of chiropractic, very few people see chiropractors, and here are some of the reasons why.

They don't know what to expect. Because most people have gone to see a medical doctor, they have an overall understanding of what to expect when they walk into the office. They expect to see a little window, to be handed some paperwork to fill out, and then eventually to visit with the doctor and tell them where it hurts. They also know that they'll likely be handed a prescription that will help their symptoms and they can be on their way.

What happens when they go to see a chiropractor? They don't really know. They assume it's similar to a visit to an MD, except that instead of being given a prescription, the chiropractor is likely to "pop" something. Do they really need something "popped?" They're not sure, so they avoid chiropractors and go with what they know.

They don't know if chiropractic care can help their condition. The most common advertisements depict chiropractors as helping with recovery after auto accidents and with low back pain, but maybe they aren't experiencing that. Maybe they have headaches or neck pain or shoulder pain. Can a chiropractor help with that? They take some time to Google it and run through some websites, discovering that some chiropractic websites state what conditions they help and some don't say much at all.

Can a chiropractor help them? Again, they're not sure, so they just go back to what they know, which is typically the medical system. They want relief and they want it fast. They've gotten relief before by getting a prescription, so once again they find themselves at their physician's office.

HOW DOES CHIROPRACTIC EDUCATION COMPARE TO MEDICAL EDUCATION?

People are often surprised to discover that the education received at a chiropractic college is quite similar to the education received in medical school. Candidates for chiropractic college must complete a minimum of three years of college-level courses prior to entering school, and completion of a doctor of chiropractic degree requires four to five years of professional coursework. Also, the education of a chiropractor is similar in total classroom hours to that of a medical doctor. See the chart below for total classroom hours for both professions. [Sources: "Chiropractic Education: A Comparison to Medical Education," MAC Journal (April 2009); Coulter, Ian, "A Comparative Study of Chiropractic and Medical Education." Alternative Therapies (September 1998), Vol. 4, No. 5; Parker Foundation, "How Well Educated is Your Chiropractor?"]

CHIROPRACTIC EDUCATION VS. MEDICAL EDUCATION		
Chiropractic	Subject	Medical
540	Anatomy – Physiology	508
240	Physiology	326
360	Pathology-Geriatrics-Pediatrics	401
165	Chemistry	325
120	Microbiology	114
630	Diagnosis, Dermatology, Ears, Eyes, Nose, Throat	324
320	Neurology	112
360	Radiology	148
60	Psychology-Psychiatry	144
60	Obstetrics-Gynecology	148
210	Orthopedics	156
3065	TOTAL	2706

HOW THE BODY HEALS

The human body is born with an intelligence that works continuously to keep us in good health. Even D.D. Palmer never actually took credit for healing ailments through chiropractic. He always regarded the body as the one that healed itself. His practices merely helped the body to do what it is completely capable of doing. As more research is done, the medical community continues to be astounded by the things that Palmer seemed to know in the late 1800s. For example, it's now been revealed that the stomach and gut area holds a second brain and how we treat that brain can heal the rest of our body. On a basic level, the systems of the whole body are intertwined in an even more complex way than we imagined; however, when it comes to alleviating its own ailments, the concept is very simple. Nerves are the central force behind the interconnectedness of systems, and alleviating them will bring relief to all.

WHAT IS INNATE INTELLIGENCE AND HOW DOES IT WORK?

The inborn intelligence that Palmer first noticed is called innate intelligence. It is with us from the moment of our birth until the moment of our death. It is always working, whether we notice it or not, much like our breathing. It keeps us alive and healthy and strives for stability both internally and externally.

Let's look at some seemingly simple things. When it's hot outside, that external environment directly affects our internal one. Our body temperature begins to rise, and our body senses this. It smartly adapts to lower our temperature back down to the normal level by causing us to sweat, which cools us. Conversely, if it's freezing cold outside, our body will respond by shivering to help warm us up.

If you go skiing and break your leg, you must go to the doctor, who will set it back in place and put a cast or boot on it to keep it from moving. Without the doctor's treatment, your bone wouldn't heal correctly; however, it is your own body that does the healing. The doctor merely aligns everything to ensure your body heals it in just the right place.

If you're a parent, you probably panic when your young children have a fever, but a fever is actually a very good thing. It's the body's innate intelligence hard at work again, fighting away the virus within it because the higher temperature kills the virus.

There are many examples of how innate intelligence functions in our bodies daily, and we never notice it. Our bodies are fascinating in that everything is communicating at all times. This communication happens from our brain to our body through numerous, tiny highways called nerves. They are the pathways to and from our brain, transporting messages all the time, back and forth from brain to body and body to brain. For our innate intelligence to keep us healthy and thriving, our nerves must be free to keep constant communication flowing through the body.

Why would our nerve messages get blocked up? Well, it doesn't take much pressure on our nerves to reduce their function. The weight of a quarter can cause nerve function to decrease by as much as 60 percent. In the spine, there are 24 vertebrae which, when in the correct position, should be flexible. With these freely moveable joints, we are able to move about and be active, which is a very good thing! The problem is that, because these 24 vertebrae move freely, they can become subluxated, misaligned, or fixated in an improper position, leading to irritation of nerve roots and causes inflammation. In addition, when the body is inflamed, this can also put pressure on the nerves, and wherever those nerves supply, that part of the body will be affected. When this happens, innate intelligence cannot work as it should. This is why chiropractic is so important for keeping the entire body healthy naturally.

CENTERING YOURSELF FOR INNATE INTELLIGENCE

As you learn more about any disease process or condition, you are likely to find that one of the always-present indicators of something being wrong in your body is too much inflammation. Reducing inflammation in your body immediately changes your health and well-being for the better. The good news is that by adding chiropractic care to your routine and making lifestyle improvements, you can take care of yourself and your own innate intelligence to help your body reduce unhealthy inflammation and function as it should.

When you engage in techniques that allow your body's innate intelligence to work as it should, you're releasing a flow of your body's natural healing energy. Although innate intelligence doesn't heal you, it is the vessel through which your body's healing begins. The process is empowering and involves each of us accepting the consequences of our lifestyles.

For example, those who do not eat healthy foods suffer from all sorts of ailments, which leads to inflammation and the impairment of innate intelligence. With a chiropractic adjustment, the pressure on the nerves is reduced, which allows the innate intelligence function to take over. However, it's not up to just chiropractors to solve your problem. If you don't take care of yourself, you'll never heal. Once you've been adjusted, eating the right things and caring for your body will allow innate intelligence to take over, sending the messages, vitamins, minerals, and other essentials to the right places in your body so that your body can heal itself.

THE INTELLIGENCE WITHIN

Our innate intelligence is something we must trust. Our bodies know themselves so well. It's like one big computer that is always running and scanning itself, alerting the brain to problems and attempting to solve them. And it is completely capable of solving these problems on its own when the flow of energy is unimpaired. If you stop and think for a moment of all the things your body is doing at this exact moment while you are reading this, it's truly overwhelming. It's like thinking about the span of the universe. It's very hard to comprehend.

However, you don't need to stress yourself out thinking of the complexities of the human body—your brain is even wired to stop you from doing so. But when your innate intelligence is compromised by impeded nerves, your body can't respond as it should; the inflammation and pressure on the nerves must be relieved. With the latest research on the brain in the gut, more and more medical professionals are finally beginning to look at chiropractic in a more positive light.

Since the late 1800s, when medicines and cures began to burst forth, it impacted people the way it still does today: we believe that we cannot get well without medicines. With chiropractic and innate intelligence, it's becoming more and more clear that clearing the blockage to the nervous system will allow the human body to do its job.

TRUSTING THE HUMAN BODY'S INNATE INTELLIGENCE

Now that you know about innate intelligence, it's imperative to accept what it can do—to trust it to heal. That's not to say that you should slice open your hand while cooking and allow yourself to bleed out. You'll still need medical treatment, perhaps some stitches. But those stitches aren't healing you. They're merely helping align the broken parts of your flesh with each other so that your body can regenerate the skin. It knows to do this through innate intelligence, sensing a breach in the skin and sending cells to rebuild it.

THE CONNECTION TO INNATE INTELLIGENCE AND YOUR SUCCESS

Because every cell in your body is connected with your innate intelligence, once you meaningfully harness this power, you can perform better in all areas of your life—even in your work. By healing your body and functioning at your most optimum level, you can perform better and be more successful. Innate intelligence is like a virus scan on your computer. It senses something and immediately responds to correct the issue—when your body is not inflamed and restricting the nerve pathways.

Your innate intelligence depends on your nervous system and its proper functionality. It sounds so simple, but the misalignment of one thing can throw off the whole body. By correcting the subluxations, chiropractic makes your nerve supply function properly. This results in zero interference, which allows your body to completely communicate with every portion of itself uninhibited.

CHANGING THE GAME FOR CHIROPRACTIC

Despite years of credible research studies and demonstrated outcomes, great bias against chiropractors still exists. Unfortunately, some chiropractors are practicing that should never be allowed to do so for lack of training. They tarnish the reputation of proper chiropractors. Despite the number of other medical doctors in other fields who lack the training and necessary credentials, these fields of medicine seem never quite as demeaned as much as chiropractic.

Other problems stem from insurance issues, which can be an intensive mess on its own for the American people. Many insurance companies only want to cover medical costs when something is healed, and true chiropractors don't heal. They merely open the pathways of the nervous system to allow the body to heal, which is a mystifying concept to many.

Add to that the stranglehold that pharmaceutical companies have on the health care industry, and it's a sad state of affairs. However, there is a silver lining: people today are looking more for natural solutions and are questioning what is actually in the foods, medicines, and supplements they're being ordered to take. By learning about how inflammation is at the root of so many maladies and seeking natural ways to treat it, they're allowing their own innate intelligence to thrive and to reignite their lives without pain or suffering.

We all deserve to live a healthy, productive life. Chiropractic is the way to open these doors for us to let the flow of our body's rhythm take over and heal the small things for which we've been overmedicating ourselves. Seeking out a truly effective chiropractor is the first step in healing so that innate intelligence may flourish. Once that happens, the body can do the miraculous things it was born to do.

PART THREE

WHAT IS FUNCTIONAL MEDICINE?

WHAT IS FUNCTIONAL MEDICINE?

The U.S. health care system spends more than 80 percent of its funds on chronic medical conditions with limited success. It's the biggest health care system in the world, amounting to more than $3 trillion per year. Although it provides public health care to around just 20 percent of the population, the rest are dependent on health insurance or paying out of pocket. Despite this spending, the U.S. lags behind most developed countries when it comes to health care.

There is undoubtedly something wrong with the current health care approach that pays enormous attention to acute conditions, relieves symptoms, and provides treatment through various specialists trying to cure the disease of each organ. Modern allopathic doctors view patients as though they are made of several independent systems.

Functional Medicine (FM) takes a different approach from allopathic. Functional medicine looks at a person as a single entity, believing that everything is interconnected. It attempts to find the root cause of the ailment, analyzes the potential triggers that led to the present condition, and pays specific attention to the patient's characteristics to provide a personalized remedy and treatment approach.

Functional medicine, the brainchild of Jeffery Bland, PhD, started emerging as one of the branches of alternative medicine in the 1980s. The foundation of functional medicine can be traced back to 1991, when the Institute of Functional Medicine (IFM) was established.

> *"Functional Medicine is a system. A biology-based approach that focuses on identifying and addressing the root cause of disease. Each symptom or differential diagnosis may be one of many contributing to an individual's illness."*
>
> – The Functional Medicine Approach, or IFM.

Functional medicine attempts to track the origin of the disease, so it pays specific attention to the patient's history. Chronic conditions start much earlier than they are felt and reported, which is something that even allopathy has begun to accept. Now, most researchers recognize that diabetes exists at least a decade before being diagnosed, and the same is true for neurodegenerative diseases. Researchers firmly agree that chronic diseases are the result of a faulty lifestyle practiced for years or even decades. Thus, chronic short duration of sleep may cause hypertension, heart attack, depression, dementia, infertility, and so on.

Despite all of the progress and understanding, allopathy rarely tries to correct the root causes, looking instead at the immediate symptoms and alterations in body functions. Thus, drugs are prescribed to control glucose when treating diabetes and antiseizure medications to keep neuropathy in check. FM is evidence-based medicine with different opinions and outlooks. It sees illness as a reaction or change that occurs due to interaction with the internal and external environments. FM attempts to identify and reverse the ill effects of that interaction by trying to rid the body of the cause and, therefore, cure the system.

Each individual is unique—living and interacting within its own microenvironment, having a unique lifestyle and influencing factors. The allopathic community understands this, though it does not often take that into consideration when trying to treat diseases. Despite an understanding of the uniqueness of patients, genetics, and environment, allopathy has a "one-size-fits-all" approach.

On the other hand, functional medicine understands that individuals' lifestyle choices and specificity of interaction with the environment play a central role in disease development, modification, and alteration of its course. Interaction with the environment may also change the behavior of the gene leading to changes in the body: *structural integrity, transport, communication, biotransformation, energy production, defense and repair, and assimilation.* **These are the seven core imbalances recognized in functional medicine.**

To assist the practicing clinicians of functional medicine, the Institute of Functional Medicine has come up with many innovative tools, including one called the **functional medicine matrix**, which helps interpret the patient better. With the help of modern research and science, it helps doctors understand the seven core imbalances, thus bridging the knowledge gap. With the help of a matrix, practitioners can better identify the underlying causes (triggers and mediators) of various chronic diseases.

Functional medicine emphasizes four vital components in clinical practice:

1. Carefully listen to and interpret the patient's narrative regarding the ailment and pay specific attention to minute details.
2. Pay attention to modifiable lifestyle factors that may be behind the illness, such as lack of exercise, nutritional deficiencies, lack of sleep, and stress.
3. Complete the matrix table for clarity of understanding of the root causes of diseases.
4. Create a doctor-patient partnership.

Let's look at an example: the doctor-patient collaboration, which is one of the most crucial principles of functional medicine. This principle of the partnership has been well studied in the chronic care model of allopathy, yet it is rarely deployed in practice. In allopathy, the doctor prescribes, and the doctor is in authority, while the patient is expected to fulfill the provided instructions. In functional medicine, the relationship is very different. The doctor and patient are partners in the treatment process.

Functional medicine is not against modern pharmaceutical drugs or allopathic medicine. It complements allopathic medicine, providing the best of various systems. Thus, functional medicine attempts to reverse disease processes through lifestyle modification, exercise, dietary changes, use of high-quality food supplementation, and even pharmacological drugs. To some extent, functional medicine can be seen as practicing something that allopathic medicine has long talked about but continues to neglect.

Consider, for example, conditions such as dementia, COPD, and diabetes. Most medical texts say that treatment should start with identifying the root cause, followed by lifestyle modification. Yet in actual practice, allopathic doctors rarely do that; instead, they immediately begin treatment with proven, or even unproven, drugs.

In functional medicine, treatment starts with fundamental changes in lifestyle, nutritional interventions, and prioritizing the correction of the seven core imbalances. In the end, it results in a better quality of life, better outcomes, and reduced costs of health care, with or without minimal use of any toxic therapies.

Another emphasis of functional medicine is on the so-called therapeutic relationship. The qualities of trust, gratitude, vulnerability, presence, humility, deep listening, reflection, and connection are considered essential to the healing process. It is vital to understand the preparedness of the patient to change. Outcomes depend significantly on the practitioner's ability to motivate patients to comply with lifestyle prescription and to make necessary changes, thus allowing the body to begin correcting underlying imbalances.

One of the greatest strengths of functional medicine is that its principles can be applied with equal success to all the disciplines and specialties of medicine. The template of the functional medicine matrix can be utilized to understand the patient and the root causes of diseases, and in planning the therapeutic approach. Functional medicine tries to combine various components of traditional and nontraditional medicine to treat, prevent, and reverse chronic diseases.

Though practitioners of allopathic medicine agree with many underlying principles of functional medicine—identifying the root cause of illness, lifestyle modifications, stress management, and nutrition therapy—most are skeptical about many tenets of functional medicine. Many practitioners of allopathy are skeptical about the methods that correct the flow of vital energy, techniques to help activate and deactivate genes during development (gene switching), and detoxification. The reason for this skepticism is often their lack of awareness and lack of understanding of some of the latest findings in research.

Most allopathic doctors would say it is not possible to switch genes on and off to cure ailments. However, those that state this forget about (or are unaware of) the field in modern science called epigenetics, the study of heritable phenotype changes that do not involve alterations in the DNA sequence. Epigenetics most often involves changes that affect gene activity and expression. Such effects on cellular and physiological phenotypic traits may result from external or environmental factors or be part of normal development. The standard definition of epigenetics requires these alterations to be heritable in the progeny of either cells or organisms. Epigenetics says that with lifestyle modification, it is possible to change gene expression. Simply stated, lifestyle changes may help to switch individual genes on and off. Moreover, the study of epigenetics (also part of allopathy) confirms that such changes can also be passed on to the next generation.

Correction of energy flow (bioenergy) is another area that may be discounted by practitioners of allopathy. However, it is something entirely supported by science. It is now well known that nerves and hormones control the functioning of every cell in our body. Without nerve supply, many cells would die immediately.

Functional medicine recommends looking at the body as a single entity, not something comprised of independent systems. Modern science is now proving that various bodily systems are more related to one another than was ever thought before. We have all heard about, and probably experienced, a "gut feeling," which occurs because our gut has more neurons than the spine, and these neurons secrete hundreds of hormones, neurohormones, and neurotransmitters. In recent years, scholars have coined the term "diffuse endocrinal system" because they realized that hormones are released by almost all the tissues and not just by the traditional endocrinal organs. It has been well proven that even fat tissue around a person's midsection secretes several hormones that a have a role in health and disease development.

Many practitioners of allopathy are also skeptical about reversing chronic ailments, even though there are many examples of this being done. Moreover, in the last couple of decades, it has been established that under specific conditions, every organ has the capacity to recover and regenerate.

Stem-cell therapy and regenerative medicine started by identifying the super-regenerative powers of particular tissues, such as bone marrow or embryonic stem cells. Now, it is recognized beyond doubt that stem cells, which can regenerate, exist in all tissues and organs.

Much of the skepticism regarding functional medicine is due to a lack of awareness and/or neglect of long-proven principles of modern health science. The diagnostic approach in functional medicine differs significantly from allopathic medicine. Functional medicine's focus is the prevention of disease by identifying the root cause, unlike allopathic medicine, where tests are usually done to confirm a diagnosis. Thus, in allopathic medicine, doctors order a test to confirm the pathological changes and diagnosis. In contrast, in functional medicine, the doctor's goal is to learn more about conditions such as leaky gut syndrome, infections, food intolerance, and hormonal and nutrient deficiencies, not just to search for some inflammatory markers that indicate a disease process.

For example, functional medicine doctors often order a comprehensive stool test to learn how the digestive system is working and about the levels of good and bad bacteria in the gut. This determines the presence of highly virulent infections, as well as how a person is absorbing various nutrients. In a blood test, doctors of functional medicine are interested in nutritional deficiencies that may lead to depression, fibromyalgia, sleep disturbances, diabetes, and fatigue, unlike allopathic doctors who are more interested in markers of inflammation and infection.

Doctors of functional medicine are also greatly interested in the complete hormonal profile. They pay attention to the adrenal stress profile, as these hormones are the most significant indicators of acute or chronic stress, which is behind the development of various diseases. Often, it is hormonal changes, chronic stress, and inflammation that lead to autoimmune disorders.

Other tests that doctors of functional medicine will order are a detailed cardiometabolic profile and tests for heavy metals and chemical toxins. Doctors of functional medicine also look deeper into food sensitivities.

So, who should consult with a doctor of functional medicine, and for what health issues and diseases does it work best?

Allopathic medicine is excellent at acute care, meaning if you were having severe pain in your abdomen along with vomiting and diarrhea, you wouldn't want to see a functional medicine doctor. You would need acute care, or you could die of your appendix rupturing. Functional medicine is about disease prevention, finding the root causes of chronic health challenges or diseases, detoxification, metabolism correction, and disease reversal.

Think about it like this: If a person had a heart attack, allopathic medicine could help to save a life, but once the condition has stabilized, functional medicine can help to identify the causes of worsening cardiac health, high blood pressure, or high cholesterol, for example; it can help to correct the faulty lifestyle and assist in disease reversal. Functional medicine can be especially helpful with the treatment of diabetes, asthma, food allergies, celiac disease, autoimmune diseases, mood disorders, and much more.

Functional medicine is for anyone who wants to get to the bottom of the disease, rather than just continue to subdue the symptoms.

In the chapters that follow, we will discuss some of the many different components of functional medicine, including our normal digestive system, diet, genetics, germs, toxins, and some potent tools that I've used to regain health and drive down inflammation.

THE BIOLOGY OF NORMAL DIGESTION

The importance of healthy digestion is crucial to our health and vitality. Our digestive system influences our immunity, detoxification, and mental health, as well as hormones. Our gut lining is a protective barrier between foods we eat and microorganisms to which we are exposed, and our immune system, which influences our reactions to foods and whether we develop food sensitivities, inflammatory conditions, and chronic diseases.

The whole digestive function consists of three primary stages:

1. the decomposition of food
2. the intake of nutrients
3. the expelling of waste substances

The upper gastrointestinal lining is responsible for decomposing the foods that we eat and absorbing nutrients. It includes our mouths, esophagus, pancreas, lower esophageal lining, and gallbladder.

Our tongue, teeth, and saliva all function synergistically to initiate the decomposition of food, which should be pureed after it leaves our mouth, not broken down into only two or three large chunks of food.

Once our mouth starts the work of digestion, we swallow it, and the food travels through the esophageal wall. The esophagus is a densely built tube that uses a movement called "peristalsis" to trigger a pattern of coordinated movements to push our food down the stomach lining. As the food travels down the esophagus, it joins with the upper edge of the stomach where the lower esophageal sphincter is found. This is the window that connects the esophagus to our stomach, and in numerous instances, this is where some problems associated with influx function occur. Conditions such as acid reflux and other digestive irregularities can start here, and many people don't realize it.

After the food travels from the esophagus to the stomach, the system begins to churn the food with stomach acid and enzymes to form a pulp named "chyme," which resembles apple cream in texture. It's an acidic puree coming from our stomach when the digestive procedure is completed. At this point, our stomach generates a substance called "intrinsic factor," which enables the proper utilization and absorption of vitamin B12. If that doesn't happen, we won't be able to absorb B12, and we can become deficient in this important nutrient. The stomach typically releases stomach acid (hydrochloric acid), and the pancreas is responsible for releasing digestive enzymes like protease, lipase, and amylase, which continue to decompose and process the food that passes through our systems.

Digestion is next handled by the gallbladder. Most people are unaware that the gallbladder has a very vital digestion role to fulfill. It deposits bile coming from the liver, which is then released to the small intestine walls as the chyme travels through. Besides depositing bile, the gallbladder also produces bile salts, which are formed to break down the fat in the food so that it gets absorbed properly. The gallbladder retains these compounds until it recognizes food that travels through with a high-fat concentration. Then it draws together and spatters the bile liquid onto the food, enabling the breakdown of fats into smaller molecules (emulsification) for our bodies to absorb and store. Therefore, if you don't have a gallbladder, you're not able to deposit bile and produce it when needed. Unfortunately, this will make digestion more difficult.

The next digestive phase is concerned with the lower gastrointestinal tract. This area is mainly accountable for absorbing and expelling the food. It's made up of the small intestine, the appendix, the ileocecal valve, the large intestine (colon), the rectum, and the anus.

Most digestive functions and absorption occur in the 10 to 20 feet (when stretched) of the small intestine. Once absorption takes place, the food travels into the lesser right quadrant, where the small intestine opens into the large intestine. This opening is called the ileocecal sphincter and is responsible for regulating the circulation of processed food from the small intestine to the colon. Both the appendix and ileocecal sphincter are located inside a small cavity that connects the small intestine with the large intestine.

The processed food then passes through the colon (large intestine), whose function is to ingest water from the stool. It harbors numerous existing bacterial cultures that make up the gut flora of your microbiome. The microbiome is the genetic material of all the microbes, including bacteria, fungi, protozoa, and viruseses, that live inside us. Healthy gut (stomach/belly) function is crucial for optimal health. Your gut is the home to 500 species and three pounds of bacteria. Maintaining a healthy flora promotes a normal ecology in the gut and allows for complete digestive function.

Especially important for our flora is the breakdown of carbohydrates, which produce substances known as short-chain fatty acids. This process is so important because short-chain fatty acids feed our flora and produce a healthier microbiome. After we have utilized the nutrients from our food, the physiological bacteria in our gut consume whatever food products are left, and the bacteria expel short-chain fatty acids, the main source of nutrition for the cells in your intestinal wall. The digestive function is then completed with the expelling of waste through our rectum and anus. It holds our stool until there is enough bulk to trigger the message to the brain to have a bowel movement.

Another vital biological aspect, even though it's not a formal part of the digestive system, is gut-associated lymphoid tissue (GALT). Our GALT forms approximately 75 percent of our immune system and envelops the intestinal lining. GALT's purpose is to protect us in case our system endures an unfortunate event, like an infection, food poisoning, or sensitivity. It also carries out an absorptive function. An adult of average build has an absorptive space equivalent to the range of a small tennis court in their intestinal lining.

COMMON DIGESTIVE IRREGULARITIES

Now that we've outlined important digestive functions, this section will be dedicated to describing the three most common digestive irregularities seen in my practice:

1. heartburn
2. dysbiosis
3. leaky gut

For those who endure heartburn/indigestion, the word "burn" is a very accurate description of how it feels. Most often we think of heartburn and/or indigestion as having so much acid in our stomach that it spills up into our esophagus. It's vital to understand that, in response to eating food, the stomach releases hydrochloric acid or HCL, which is the primary gastric acid secreted by the stomach. However, if we've undergone any of the following, our stomach's ability to produce the necessary HCL may be hindered.

- increased amounts of stress
- adrenal fatigue
- immune system dysfunction (invaded by specific viruses or bacteria)

- overuse of antacids
- an overloaded system due to poor eating habits
- advancing age
- other chronic diseases

It may seem counterintuitive to say that having too little stomach acid would cause a burning sensation in our throats. Let me explain. As our stomach becomes burdened by the above-mentioned conditions, we lose our ability to produce sufficient HCL; therefore, our food cannot be thoroughly digested. When our food isn't thoroughly digested, it putrefies, and the acidic by-products come splashing back up into the esophagus, causing the acidic burning sensation commonly known as heartburn or indigestion.

Problems with our pancreas can also lead to indigestion. The pancreas secretes digestive enzymes that can also be affected by the above-mentioned conditions. When this happens, pancreatic activity can slow way down. When the ability of our pancreas to secrete enzymes is depressed, the stomach is pressured to release more acid in order to properly break down the food. This overload of stomach acid production leads to poor digestion (maldigestion), which means our food is not digested thoroughly. This progression of insufficient digestion triggers symptoms like gas, belching, and reflux. This is one of the triggers of gastroesophageal reflux disorder, or GERD syndrome. In the cases described above, the typical course of treatment is to diminish the acid in the stomach. Whether you have too much or too little acid, the result feels the same: the uncomfortable, burning sensation we call GERD/heartburn/

indigestion. The bigger problem occurs when we take medication to reduce the acid, which then leaves us with nothing to digest and break down our food, furthering this vicious cycle of digestive dysfunction.

Another very common digestive irregularity is dysbiosis, which affects nearly all of us at different points in our life. Dysbiosis occurs when there's an imbalance of beneficial vs. bad bacteria (the bad bugs outnumber the good bugs) inside our gut. Imagine dysbiosis as your front yard filled with weeds that cover the weakened grass. You can't have a nice, green, robust pasture when it's infested with too many weeds and lacks sufficient amounts of healthy grass. However, if the grass is healthy and full enough, weeds can't take over. If the distribution of weeds vs. healthy grass gets out of proportion, dysbiosis happens. Many factors contribute to dysbiosis, including bacterial infections, yeast overgrowth, overuse of antibiotics, viruses, fungi, worms, parasites, and destructive bacteria like H. pylori, which leads to ulcers. Improper stomach digestion can also trigger this situation. If our system isn't digesting meals properly inside the stomach, the food won't have been thoroughly digested, which leads to dysbiosis. This vicious cycle will lead to more digestive dysfunction.

Leaky gut is another digestive disorder. In a healthy gut, the lining is made up of tightly connected junctions between cells in the intestinal tract. These tight junctions are perfectly spaced to allow nutrients to pass through the gut barrier into the bloodstream where we absorb them for nutrition. It also prevents large undigested proteins from getting into the bloodstream, which can be detrimental to our health. We develop a "leaky gut" when the gut barrier breaks down and the tight junctions are no longer tight (like a chain-link fence that's been busted and now has holes that allow foreign invaders to enter). The immune system perceives these large undigested proteins as a toxic substance rather than a food or a nutrient. Next, antibodies are generated that fight the protein, triggering an immune reaction.

This whole process primarily develops in the small intestine. When it occurs, it causes cellular destruction of the gut lining, resulting in high levels of inflammation that spread to other nearby areas, and gut permeability levels rises, which is why the syndrome is called "leaky gut."

If our gut area becomes hyperpermeable (or "leaky") due to gastrointestinal dysfunction triggered by intolerance and/or the entrance of an external compound into our system, our body will be subject to endemic and major toxic buildup.

GLUTEN AND ITS IMPLICATIONS FOR THE GUT AND OUR HEALTH

Gluten is a sticky protein found in wheat and other grains like rye and barley.

As noted, the gut's function is to absorb nutrients through the cell membrane into very small molecules that are then absorbed into the bloodstream and used for our benefit. These cells that line the intestinal wall are also the same cells that maintain gut permeability (the proper function of allowing nutrients to pass through but keeping others out).

In sensitive people, gluten causes the gut cells to release zonulin, which causes a leak by breaking the tight junctions apart. This leak provides unhindered entry of various toxins, microbes, and undigested food particles from the intestines into the bloodstream.

Gluten intolerance consists of two types of disorders:

1. autoimmune celiac disease
2. non-celiac gluten sensitivity (NCGS)

Studies have proven that in NCGS, when gluten-related peptides enter the bloodstream, they cause extraintestinal manifestations such as ataxia, neuropathy, and encephalopathy. Gluten is also associated with psychiatric disorders such as depression, anxiety, autism, and schizophrenia in patients with NCGS. A recent study reveals that psychosis might also be a manifestation of NCGS. A gluten-free diet seems to be the safest, most effective way of treating celiac disease and NCGS.

GLUTEN INTOLERANCE: AN AUTOIMMUNE DISORDER

What's the link between autoimmune disease and gluten sensitivity? When considering autoimmune disease of the thyroid malfunctions, the joints, or even the pancreas, too often people assume that they're all totally separate disorders that share nothing in common with gluten and autoimmunity. However, these diseases have one major common denominator—the immune system. When the body starts to fight its own tissue and cells, that's when autoimmune disease begins. The function of the immune system is to fight external intruders that can damage your system, not its own tissue, but this is exactly what happens once an autoimmune reaction is triggered.

Traditionally, gluten is defined as a cohesive, elastic protein that is left behind after starch is washed away from a wheat flour dough. Only wheat is considered to have true gluten. Gluten is actually made up of many different proteins, of which there are two main groups: gliadins and the glutenin (gliadin is the water-insoluble component of gluten, and glutenin is water-soluble).

Gluten sensitivity/intolerance is an autoimmune disorder that triggers a series of inflammatory cascades in the system and leads to numerous health issues, including heart diseases, brain problems, bone and joint problems, skin problems, and many others. In other words, a person is gluten intolerant when their system triggers an antigen response to gluten.

Every time you eat something that contains gluten (bread, pasta, most packaged foods), large, undigested proteins are exposed to your immune system, causing your immune function to attack them. You then generate IgE antibodies, which are deemed scientifically as a food allergy, and your system can generate other antibodies too, like IgG or IgA, which are usually considered food intolerances or food sensitivities. In their mechanic nature, both food allergies and food intolerances/ sensitivities essentially function in the same manner. They trigger inflammation inside your body at various speeds but identical in their activity. It's just their antibodies that are different, but can have life-threatening consequences in the case of a food allergy.

If you recall the previous discussion on leaky gut syndrome, this mechanism is identical. Proteins that "leak" in through our too-porous gut are exposed to our immune system repeatedly, which may lead to immune challenges (autoimmune diseases). These proteins contain only a specific amino-acid sequence, and when our bodies are inappropriately exposed to them on a regular basis, we begin to experience what's called "molecular mimicry," where proteins exposed to our immune system have the same amino-acid pattern as the proteins naturally found in our body. This is how autoimmunity begins. When our body's immune system has been assaulted enough, this switch is flipped on and our immune system targets the protein(s) that entered the body externally.

When such an interaction occurs, our system activates a series of immune reactions against our own body's tissues. This is considered an autoimmune disorder (self-destroying disorder). If we continue exposing our system to these proteins, it will continue reacting and generating antibodies to fight our own tissues.

Having an allergy or sensitivity to gluten is not the same as having an autoimmune disorder. Through a stool or genetic test, you may learn that you have the genes for gluten sensitivity. Even though you could bear a gene for gluten sensitivity, it may not be activated in your system. If the gene isn't activated, there will be no autoimmune reaction to gluten.

Many people have been tested and discovered that they carry the gene, but it wasn't activated yet. The issue is that many circumstances could activate such a gene. Physical or emotional trauma and stress, which are totally irrelevant to gluten, can switch on the gene. Moreover, a stressed, overburdened immune system can also activate these genes. This is why some people noticed more digestive issues after a particularly stressful event or illness.

If tests show that you have autoimmunity and bear the gene for gluten intolerance, it's wise to avoid eating gluten altogether. Because it's an autoimmune disorder, every time you consume gluten, it's attacking your system and brain composition (gut-brain connection), even though you may not experience any outer symptoms. You're essentially giving yourself internal inflammation when you eat foods you're sensitive to and in the case of an allergy, this can lead to anaphylaxis. Gluten induces a fight against opiate receptors in the brain and overexcites them, which may lead to anxiety/depression, attention deficit hyperactivity disorder, autism, and other mental health issues. Multiple studies validate that if you have this disorder and consume a small amount of gluten, you could be destroying long-term health.

If you have autoimmunity and the gene for gluten sensitivity, there is a high risk that your children will inherit this gene as well. Making your child aware of this matter early on, before any negative health symptoms become apparent, will pay dividends in their health in the long term. Remember, it's not only a matter of outer symptoms. If you carry the gene, any exposure to gluten/gliadin will wreak havoc on your gut, immune system, and brain. Prevention is the key to long-term health, regardless of your age.

Autoimmunity, in a few words, implies that your own immune system is fighting your own cells. This is the common denominator that contributes to the formation of health problems. When the immune disorders are considered together as a single issue, they are the third prevailing cause of death in the U.S., which is an impressive figure. With the strong link between immune disorders and gluten intolerance, it's an extremely important correlation that needs to be acknowledged before it's too late.

GLUTEN SENSITIVITY: AN UNDERDIAGNOSED WIDESPREAD ISSUE

It was once believed that gluten sensitivity mostly affected children and caused symptoms such as diarrhea, weight loss, and the inability to grow tall. Today, however, we're aware that people of all ages can suffer from gluten sensitivity.

Not everyone has a problem with gluten sensitivity, but it is more widespread than most of us realize because issues with gluten sensitivity are commonly undiagnosed or misdiagnosed. The issue is more predominant in people who have a long-term illness. The most critical kind of gluten sensitivity is celiac disease, which affects 1 percent of people in the U.S. (around 3 million Americans), the majority of whom haven't been properly diagnosed and are unaware they have it. Less serious forms of gluten sensitivity occur more frequently and affect approximately 30 percent of the general population.

The typical celiac patient tends to suffer with the symptoms of the disorder for a minimum of 10 years before they receive a proper diagnosis. They often face degrading integrity of their gut lining, unnecessary weight loss or obesity, and a malnourished body during this process. Many people I've treated over the years are concerned that something more serious is going on, but they're relieved to know that a necessary adjustment to their eating habits can restore their health and energy back to optimal levels.

Unfortunately, many people with gluten sensitivity don't have symptoms and are unaware they have an issue. Adding fuel to the fire, many doctors neglect or fail to recognize any signs of gluten sensitivity, which leads to a lack of diagnosis or misdiagnosis.

THE LINK BETWEEN GLUTEN AND YOUR HEALTH

Gluten Sensitivity

There is growing evidence that gluten intolerance is less of a fad than we thought. In fact, this infamous protein can wreak havoc on a person's bodily systems and general health. Unfortunately, many people consume ordinary foods every day that contain this protein, unaware of the adverse reactions gluten has on their systems. Anyone who chooses to munch daily on a burger, fries, and a soda is shortening their lifespan, but even if they have a big slice of whole-wheat bread instead (a healthier option), there can still be negative consequences.

Wheat and other cereals like rye, barley, spelt, and oats, as well as processed and boxed meals, contain gluten. In the average Western diet, it's also found in bread, pizzas, pies, and pasta. Furthermore, the types of wheat found in the U.S. are fortified with higher levels of gluten to make bread and bread-like products fluffy and puffy.

Gluten has been a component of human nutrition for ages. It gives us the energy and stamina we need to go through the day, and it makes us feel fuller and happier. The question that should be asked, then, is this: Why do so many of us have gluten intolerance if this is what we've been consuming every day for years? There are numerous reasons for this, including genetic predisposition and, specifically, an insufficient ability to metabolize grains and grass. Wheat first entered Europe during the medieval times, and 30 percent of European ancestors are genetically predisposed to celiac disease, which raises the risk of developing a health issue because of gluten consumption.

More of the healthier foods we consume can contain gluten, including corn and oatmeal. Not only that, it's also found in product ingredients like malt and maltodextrin, which is why reading product labels is so important.

The most shocking evidence, though, is that 99 percent of people with a gluten intolerance are unaware they have it, so they fail to blame their poor health on their gluten intolerance. As someone who works with people daily to address and improve their health concerns, this is very disappointing and challenging because the symptoms that come from gluten intolerance are 100 percent treatable.

Gluten intolerance is typically connected with two triggers: genetic predisposition and leaky gut. In the first case, being gluten sensitive does not imply that you are a sensitive person. It just means that your DNA and immune system are unable to tolerate gluten. Your immune system may falsely flag it as a foreign intruder and attempt to attack it. In essence, this is what "gluten sensitivity" means. Fortunately, you can easily be tested for gluten sensitivity and learn whether you have these genetic tendencies.

THE IMPACT OF GLUTEN SENSITIVITY

Americans' health pays a big price due to the sneaky way gluten infiltrates our foods and affects our bodies. Undiagnosed gluten sensitivities burden the health care system, driving up health care costs. Doctors at Sigma Health Care (Australia's leading pharmacy network) examined 10 million patients and realized that those who were accurately diagnosed with celiac disorder used fewer health care services and decreased medical expenses by more than 30 percent. The issue is, just a mere 1 percent of the people suffering from celiac disease get diagnosed accurately. That implies that 99 percent of the population living with this disorder don't realize it. This burdens the medical system and costs us millions of dollars each year.

Gluten imposes serious physiological effects on people. Research published in the *Journal of the American Medical Association* (JAMA) studying two groups of people who were either diagnosed or not diagnosed, showed that those with inactive celiac disease or gluten intolerance had an elevated risk of death, mainly due to heart problems and cancer. This research considered 30,000 patients from 1969 to 2008 and examined deaths in three control groups:

- patients with fully developed celiac disease
- those with intestinal inflammation but not completely developed celiac disease
- those with a completely full-blown disease, which implies they had increased gluten antibodies yet a non-positive intestinal biopsy

In a shocking revelation, the study found that patients who experienced celiac disorder had a 39 percent elevated risk of death, while people with gut inflammation linked to gluten intolerance had a 72 percent elevated risk of death. Those who had a mild gluten intolerance, but not celiac disease, showed a 35 percent elevated risk. This shocking finding demonstrates that one doesn't have to suffer from a full-blown celiac disorder with a positive intestinal test to be impacted by gluten intolerance. Despite what many believe, milder levels of gluten sensitivity also trigger major health issues and side effects.

We should also point out that, worldwide, there has been a 400 percent increase in the development of heart disease and cancer since a half century ago. However, little to no attention has been paid to the rapid rise of celiac disease.

Because gluten sensitivity has an impact on the body's immune system, inflammation can occur in countless ways. Celiac disease and gluten intolerance conceal numerous other health issues and disorders of various kinds. A literature review report published in the *New England Journal of Medicine* numbered over fifty disorders linked to gluten sensitivity, including arthritis, osteoporosis, lupus, rheumatoid arthritis, irritable bowel syndrome, inflammatory bowel disorder, multiple sclerosis, cancer, anemia, adrenal fatigue, and nearly all autoimmune diseases. Gluten intolerance is associated with diabetes, asthma, psoriasis, eczema, poor thyroid function, lupus, dermatitis, and Sjögren's syndrome, an automimmune disease that attacks the glands that make tears and saliva. It is also linked to many mental health problems and nervous system disorders such as depression, anxiety, epilepsy, schizophrenia, headaches, migraines, and nerve impairment. It has even been connected to the onset of autism. Failing to diagnose celiac disease or even gluten intolerance can cause suffering and even death (indirectly) for millions of people.

GLUTEN SENSITIVITY AND LEAKY GUT SYNDROME

It has been demonstrated that in someone who experiences gluten sensitivity, the system flags gluten as a foreign intruder, perceiving it as a toxic substance rather than a food or a nutrient—in other words, as with an autoimmune disease. The immune system generates antibodies that fight gluten/gliadin. This process primarily occurs in the small intestine where the destruction takes place, which causes high levels of inflammation that spread to other nearby areas as gut permeability levels rise. This syndrome is called "leaky gut." When the intestine gets leaky, antibodies can break free from the small intestine and enter the bloodstream.

Gluten is a form of protein, and bountiful proteins exist in our system. Once these antibodies break free from the small intestine and flow throughout the bloodstream, components of our system's protein makeup are very similar to gluten's protein format. Eventually, a disarray occurs, known as "crossed reactivity." Antibodies trigger a fight against our body's cells, setting up an autoimmune disorder. Furthermore, these antibodies break away from the small intestine and become incorporated into the general blood flow of the system. The antibodies start fighting the body's cells because they're disoriented. They assume these are gluten when, in reality, they aren't.

The other function related to gluten sensitivity concerns the body's adrenal glands, also known as the body's "stress glands." As the adrenal glands lose their function (which occurs due to numerous chronic issues that can happen in the body), they can produce the wrong amounts of cortisol. Despite cortisol getting a bad rap as the fat-storage hormone, it actually plays many important roles in keeping our body healthy. Cortisol is mainly responsible for keeping our immune function under control, so that it only triggers a fight only when it's needed.

Unfortunately, when the adrenal glands are chronically overworked, they begin to lose function and are unable to secrete the necessary hormones, which suppresses the immune system, agitating and overexciting it and triggering a fight. This is another situation where our body is affected by autoimmune disease.

This situation is also found, to a lesser degree, in allergies. Those who suffer from adult-activated allergies (adults who have no prior history/record of bee-pollen sensitivity or other allergens in the atmosphere) are affected because of spikes in their adrenal function. Suddenly, they start responding to various allergens in the atmosphere with which they previously never had issues.

Is some studies, close family members of those with gluten sensitivity have elevated chances of experiencing autoimmune disorders. It's assumed that maybe these asymptomatic relatives most likely had gluten sensitivity; however, they didn't show or feel any outward digestive symptoms, so the medical profession excluded them from the celiac disease category. This is a dangerous misconception, as it's been found that only 30 percent of gluten sensitive individuals feel any digestive symptoms. The remainder of gluten-sensitive people feel nothing. Even if a person doesn't have digestive symptoms, that does not exclude sensitivity to gluten. This is vital information, as autoimmune disorders are the third-leading cause of death in the country and cost our health care system millions of dollars each year.

GLUTEN SENSITIVITY AND OBESITY

Gluten/gliadin sensitivity can cause weight issues. Think about this: the total scope of the small intestine is almost the size of a small tennis court. When stretched it is 23 feet long. Because of the inflammation triggered by gluten, nutrients from food cannot get absorbed properly. The small intestine is specifically wired to facilitate the absorption of nutrients, releasing them into the bloodstream and then transferring them to the cells of the body. This offers the cells their fuel source to carry out their vital functions within the organism. When this process is disturbed, the cells aren't nourished with the nutrients and energy needed, and the body's cells become deficient. Food is still being taken in through our mouth, but it's not able to reach the cells and nourish the body.

Over time, our bodies become deficient in and deprived of critical nutrients and respond by slowing down our metabolic function, which leads to a slower, less efficient metabolism. Even though we aren't eating excessive amounts of food, we can end up with a weight issue. It's what we are eating that makes us overweight.

Gluten sensitivity can also influence adrenal glands to produce excessive amounts of cortisol, which can cause weight problems in patients as well. As formerly stated, gluten sensitivity and gut inflammation go hand in hand. The adrenal glands, in reaction to this inflammation, produce higher amounts of cortisol, which leads to increased amounts of body fat—in particular, belly fat and fat stored in midbody regions. This kind of fat is quite resistant to exercise and a low-calorie diet. Many people become annoyed with midbody weight gain because, despite their vigorous attempts to shed these pesky pounds, they never see any obvious difference. It's the gluten-triggered inflammation and the adrenal glands' overreaction that causes the resistant, excessive abdominal fat.

Another implication of gluten sensitivity and its effect on our adrenal system is elevated fatigue. When the adrenal glands are chronically overstimulated, our sleep quality is disturbed. Many factors can affect our circadian rhythm but eating gluten-containing foods at night can cause an elevated cortisol peak at night, which leads to poor-quality sleep. If we don't get a full, deep sleep, we'll simply gain body fat. This leads to a vicious cycle of inactivity, since if we feel tired and stressed, we won't easily exercise to shed any excess weight.

GLUTEN SENSITIVITY AND THYROID CONNECTION

One final aspect of gluten sensitivity we'll cover is the burden placed on the thyroid gland when someone eats gluten. The thyroid and adrenal glands are siblings and belong to the same region in your endocrine system, which is why I felt called to offer wellness blood testing in our office.

When there's an autoimmune reaction due to gluten/gliadin in our system, thyroid activity is affected. Our thyroid gland determines our metabolic rate, which is just one of the factors that come into play when it comes to our body's ability to burn body fat.

Although patients were presenting with concerns regarding gluten, diet, and altered thyroid activity, they weren't getting questions answered nor getting proper diagnoses. Many of them began reading voraciously on the Internet about the possible connections among diet, gluten, and thyroid function. In conventional medical practice, it's accepted that patients most likely don't have issues with gluten unless they are visibly underweight and undernourished, but that assumption couldn't be farther from the truth.

Many patients were prescribed typical medications for thyroid syndrome. It's very important that gluten-free thyroid medications are prescribed. Cytomel and various generic brands of levothyroxine are **not** gluten-free. The following are gluten free:

- armor
- synthroid
- levothyroxine (Lannet, Mylan brands only)
- levoxyl
- tirosint
- WP Thyroid (formerly Westhroid Pure)

There are various types of thyroid dysfunctions. For instance, there may be a mix of low and high thyroid function diagnosed by having specific thyroid antibodies show up as positive on lab tests. This is known as Hashimoto's thyroiditis, which is not only the most common form of thyroiditis but also the most common thyroid disorder in our country. A higher-than-normal thyroid function from an overactive thyroid is known as Graves' disease. Autoimmune disorders, such as Hashimoto's and Graves', are rooted in the immune system, which technical means they're not problems with the thyroid gland itself. Additionally, there's a close link between these disorders and people who are gluten intolerant.

Research tells us that an estimated 20 million Americans have some form of thyroid disease. In a specific trial with over 5,000 children subjects, it was discovered that 26 percent of them had gluten sensitivity and that they had thyroid antibodies present. This implies that their immune systems were fighting their own thyroid, which by definition, is Hashimoto's thyroiditis (an autoimmune disorder). Only two children of the 26 percent studied demonstrated hypothyroidism in blood tests. The major take-away in this study is that children need to be checked early on for gluten sensitivity, in the hopes of avoiding the development of a thyroid disorder.

Another research study showed that 40 percent of gluten-sensitive adults also suffered from thyroid problems. From what we've seen, once the immune system gets involved and begins to affect the thyroid gland's normal activity, it become more difficult to avoid thyroid medications or come off thyroid medications if you've been on them for any amount of time.

When you have a confirmed thyroid disorder, the wisest thing you can do is work with a functional medicine practitioner whom you trust. This person can help you navigate the waters of new dietary choices and avoid all the foods that will irritate the thyroid gland (gluten, soy, and iodine being just a few). It's also important to have your children tested because there's a high probability that they will also have the disorder. An effective treatment plan and new approach to health will assist in improved nutrient absorption and help the thyroid medications work better, which means less medication is needed to control your thyroid. In the long run, you and your family will be more likely to avoid the onset of any new autoimmune diseases that could develop in your body at a later time.

If you have an autoimmune disease and you're concerned about the development of additional autoimmune disorders, your best strategy is to significantly clean up your diet, especially avoiding gluten. Keeping these destructive proteins out of your diet helps your small intestine heal and rejuvenate. Many of our patients who have a gluten sensitivity can control or entirely reverse their autoimmune disorders when they stay away from gluten-containing food products. Moreover, someone who's attempting to avoid gluten can also prevent the onset of an inflammatory response in the gut, which reduces the chances of the development of an autoimmune disorder later in life.

IDENTIFYING GLUTEN SENSITIVITY ON YOUR OWN VS. A DOCTOR

One of the simplest ways to determine if you have a gluten sensitivity is by eliminating it from your diet entirely for three weeks. In that time, you may notice less of the more common symptoms, such as gas, bloating, irritable bowel, joint swelling, brain fog, and fatigue. During this time, it's critical to read labels to ensure that you completely avoid anything that contains gluten—including any hidden gluten in certain foods. After this trial period you can consume gluten (carefully having it for one meal and not all day long) and see if anything changes or if any symptoms reappear. If any of your symptoms become worse or you generally feel worse, avoiding gluten entirely is necessary.

There are other ways, though, to find out whether you suffer from gluten sensitivity, including medical or functional testing. This type of testing involves checking the blood for gluten and other similar antibodies.

When someone goes to the doctor to get a diagnosis of gluten intolerance, most people turn to conventional medicine. The problem with this approach is that many times it's falsely assumed that a gluten-sensitive individual will show some GI symptoms or other signs, which is a total misconception. As matter of fact, half the individuals who suffer from the most serious kind of gluten sensitivity (known as "celiac sprue") don't display any signs of typical gastrointestinal symptoms, including gas, bloating, and diarrhea.

How can this be? This changes our perspective, noting that gluten sensitivity is not a true gastrointestinal concern but an immune-system concern.

To reiterate an earlier point, you may have zero symptoms and no response to gluten when you eat it, but that does not mean you're in the clear. You may not be! Many patients are unaware that the only way to truly know if gluten is an issue for their system is to run specific tests on the immune system's activity and other tests that show whether the body is under an immunological attack. Contrary to what most people think, those who feel some signs are very fortunate because they can be diagnosed, treated, and healed early on.

Approximately one in three people feel some negative symptoms when eating gluten. This is good news! These people are the lucky ones because they can do something about their symptoms and prevent further damage. The other 70 percent of people consuming gluten don't have symptoms and therefore are unaware they could be dealing with this pressing issue.

Realistically, gluten is not the only trigger for everyone's health issues. Still, it is a major issue for a lot of people. Many of our patients' primary care physicians have told them that if they're not showing any signs of gluten sensitivity, they don't have to deal with it. This is very discouraging. Our health care system seems to be focused on the misconception that if someone doesn't display outer symptoms of gluten sensitivity, then they most likely don't have it. As a result, various health problems can be triggered, including multiple sclerosis, neuropathy, rheumatoid arthritis, and other autoimmune diseases that may take several years to develop and spread.

Unfortunately, we look at many typical health disorders this way. There are silent killer diseases, like some forms of cancer, which only present their devastating effects during the final stages of the disease. This applies to tooth decay as well: you never pay attention unless a tooth starts to ache, but by the time the tooth hurts, the decay has been there for months or even years. Pain and other symptoms are not necessarily a good indicator of how healthy we are.

The only accurate method to find out whether someone is gluten sensitive is to test them for it. We must change the way we look at our health and not fall into the trap of thinking that just because we feel healthy, we are. If we eat gluten and develop symptoms, that is fortunate. Symptoms help us prevent and avoid future health complications by acting early to address them.

TREATMENT OF GLUTEN SENSITIVITY

To treat and recover from gluten intolerance, obviously, you must eliminate gluten from your diet. Because gluten sensitivity could be the secret trigger for numerous health problems, this is a crucial first step. You still may have autoimmunity for other health issues that may not be directly connected to gluten, so paying close attention and journaling all your symptoms during this time is crucial. A great deal of the health issues we have been discussing can be difficult to identify, but the most appropriate treatment option in the case of gluten is to completely refrain from consuming gluten and all gluten-containing products.

When starting on a gluten-free lifestyle, one of the best ways to ensure success is to have helpful resources. (Please refer to the Appendices or go to www.keoughchiropractic.com for a whole host of wonderful places to turn for gluten-free eating and celiac support.)

A gluten-free diet has become so popular that many companies have a gluten-free option for the products found on grocery store shelves. Be aware, however, that "gluten-free" doesn't necessarily mean "healthy." These buzz words have been used to push products that may or may not be good for us, which is why it's very important to know if the "gluten-free grains" you're buying are, in fact, a healthy option for you and your family. The following are the top nine gluten-free grains I recommend for my patients who can tolerate grains (these can also be used as gluten-free flour for baking), and they are easily interchangeable with wheat- and gluten-containing flours:

- amaranth
- brown rice
- buckwheat
- corn grits
- millet
- oats
- quinoa
- sorghum
- teff

These foods are naturally gluten-free; however, because they may be processed and manufactured in plants where gluten-containing foods are also found, the risk of contamination goes up. It's wise to read labels closely when you've decided to eliminate gluten from your diet. The gluten-containing grains are rye, barley, and wheat, and they can be found in just about everything, including breads, pastas, soups, baked goods, cereals, sauces, and even salad dressings. You also want to avoid hidden ingredients, such as malt or maltodextrin, because those are fancy names for gluten as well.

Getting started with a gluten-free eating plan can be an overwhelming, daunting task, but the health benefits you'll experience in the long run are worth it. In fact, after being gluten-free for as little as three weeks, our patients report more energy, weight loss, less brain fog, less skin irritation, less gas and bloating, and the list goes on. The good news is you won't starve, and there are plenty of delicious, healthy options to eat and drink on your list of approved foods.

A lot of us have been programmed to eat grains multiple times a day, mainly because our original food pyramid contained loads of grains at the bottom of the pyramid. I'm often asked how eating gluten-free could possibly affect our weight. Here's the answer: eating grains (carbs) causes our body to produce insulin, which then triggers the production of fat storage. Reducing our carbohydrate intake to vegetables and other healthy, non-gluten-containing carbohydrates reduces the insulin, which then causes us to burn body fat.

In some cases, people are underweight due to gluten sensitivity. These are the hardest patients to convince that going to a gluten-free eating style won't cause them to lose additional weight. In reality, the opposite is true. Eating gluten-free will allow your gut to heal and rejuvenate, which allows for improved nutrient absorption and healthy weight management.

Remember, a gluten-free diet isn't some extreme diet of starvation, and it doesn't lack rich nutrients. It's one of the healthiest ways to feed your family and yourself. There is, of course, a trial-and-error period as there is with anything else, but you just need to keep working at it and don't give up—even if you fall off the wagon once in a while. As a side note, don't do this alone (if possible). If you're gluten sensitive/intolerant but your family isn't, have them join with you, as much as possible. You'll be doing them a favor. Likewise, if one of your children is gluten sensitive, have the entire family adopt this way of eating together. You'll all benefit in the end.

In the next section, I offer some useful tips you can follow if you suffer from gluten sensitivity that will boost your gastrointestinal health.

TIPS FOR BOOSTING GI HEALTH

Besides following a gluten-free diet, if you're suffering from gluten sensitivity, there are also some specific foods you can eat, tasks you can do, and suggestions you can implement to control gastrointestinal (GI) problems.

Tip 1: Take Your Time to Chew

It's vital to chew your food properly before you swallow it. Take breaths between your bites and aim to eat in a stress-free environment. Don't rush when you eat, take some time to chew everything properly, and let your system digest it more easily. Don't use antacids! Instead, use digestive enzymes, which are best taken in the middle of meals to assist in breaking down your food.

Tip 2: Drink Plenty of Water

Get plenty of pure, filtered water. (I love my Berkey water filtration system.) Many people don't get an adequate amount of water daily. You may be wondering how much water you should be drinking. There's a simple formula to figure it out:

divide your body weight by two. The answer to that problem is equal to the number of ounces of water you should drink daily. Although this a great rule of thumb in most cases, there are some instances when you need to change this slightly: don't drink in excess and try not to drink all your water paired with your meals because this dilutes digestive action.

Regarding water intake, many sources suggest that if you drink caffeine, you should drink that much more water in a day. For example, if you drink sixteen ounces of caffeine each morning, you must add sixteen additional ounces of water because of caffeine's diuretic effects.

Tip 3: Consume Adequate Amounts of Fiber

The average person should take in around 30 to 40 grams of fiber daily. Certain foods that are rich in fiber are the best sources of prebiotics (a type of fiber that the human body cannot digest), which have been known to improve gut health. You can get your dietary fiber from various foods like fruits, vegetables, legumes, or nuts. Try to consume a nice variety of fiber-rich foods. This will help boost the healthy cultures in your GI tract.

Tip 4: Stay Away from Sugar

Sugar feeds the spread of yeast in the body (Candida albicans) because it nourishes the naturally existing yeast in the system and "grows" weeds. It creates an imbalanced environment of intestinal bacterial overgrowth and leads to insufficient levels of vitamin B and an insufficient release of fatty acids. It also causes pH disturbance and can cause gas and bloating. (Note: "pH" stands for power of hydrogen, which is a measurement of the hydrogen ion concentration in the body. The total pH scale ranges from 1 to 14, with 7 considered neutral. A pH less than 7 is said to be acidic, and solutions with a pH greater than 7 are basic or alkaline.)

Tip 5: Refrain from Taking Prophylactic Antibiotics

I'm not advocating a complete avoidance of all kinds of antibiotics. What I'm referring to is the avoidance of prophylactic antibiotics. Additionally, it's wise to avoid taking antibiotics when they're recommended as a way to "cover all bases" when your provider isn't sure whether your issue is being caused by a bacteria or a virus. Educate yourself thoroughly on the issue at hand to understand if antibiotics are absolutely necessary before you or your children take them.

Antibiotics generally eradicate natural and beneficial bacteria in the body (which is they're called "*anti*biotics"). They attack life forms and terminate active organisms, including the beneficial bacteria found in our body, in particular, our microbiome. They may also initiate the spread of fungi like yeast and candida, which aren't eradicated by antibiotics. If you have a fungal infection, taking antibiotics isn't going to terminate it. In fact, if you don't take the proper steps to rebuild your microbiome after taking antibiotics, fungal infections may spread throughout your intestinal tract and eventually throughout your body.

Taking antibiotics frequently can also create antibiotic resistance among the bacteria that naturally live inside us, but this isn't the biggest problem. Genes inside our bacteria that make up our microbiome (the bacterial organisms in our internal and external environment that protect us from pathogens, break down food, and produce vitamins) can be switched on and become immune to antibiotics. It has been shown that this can alter the DNA of other surrounding gut bacteria and offer antibiotic immunity or resistance to the rest of the bacteria in our microbiome. This is how superbugs are created and why we have so many cases of antibiotic-resistant bugs.

Tip 6: Stay Away from Food Allergens

Food allergies or intolerances promote gut inflammation, and people tend to be the most reactive to milk, eggs, fish, crustacean shellfish, tree nuts, peanuts, wheat, and soy. There are tests to confirm such allergens through the presence of IgE or IgG antibodies and even DNA tests. I always recommend getting food-allergy testing so that you can become aware of the foods that may be harming your body and perpetuating inflammation.

Tip 7: Taking Probiotics

Probiotics are live bacteria that form the normal cultures that reside in our gut. They're the good guys in the bacterial community, and we want these to make up the majority of our gut bacteria. By supplementing with probiotics, we can help restore our health by balancing out the bacteria in our gut. Probiotics are typically available in supplement form and in some specialty foods. You can find probiotics in other forms, such as tinctures, capsules, powders, gel caps, and platelets. They can also be found in cultured foods, such as kefir, yogurt, sauerkraut, kvass, pickles kimchi, apple cider vinegar, and kombucha, to name a few. Whatever form you desire, it's available.

Years ago, people consumed cultured/fermented foods that were naturally rich in probiotics. However, since fermented foods aren't as easily accessible today, people consume them as supplements or anywhere they can squeeze them in as a snack or meal. Having a happy, balanced digestive system with the appropriate bacterial balance can eliminate gas, irritable bowel symptoms, nausea, indigestion, and many other issues affecting the gut.

Make sure you pay attention to your body after starting probiotic supplements or foods because they can sometimes make you worse. Make sure you use high-quality supplements and foods and start slow. Work up to making probiotics part of your daily intake.

Tip 8: Getting Prebiotics

Prebiotics are not the same as probiotics. Prebiotics actually nourish the probiotics and are derived from specific foods like psyllium husk, pectin, Jerusalem artichoke, and sweet potatoes. They are typically processed by the physiological flora or cultured into short-chain fatty acids (SCFA). They nourish the cells that make up the digestive lining. When someone consumes good sources of pulp like fruits and vegetables, these get fermented into prebiotics. There's no need to take them as supplements separately; just incorporate them into your regular daily diet.

Tip 9 : Have a Bowel Movement at Least Once Daily

Ideally, you should move your bowels approximately a half hour to an hour after every meal you eat, which some people may perceive as diarrhea. It isn't. Our systems are wired to function this way. The stomach expands when we eat something, which sends a nerve signal to the intestines to begin the contractions to work to expel what you've just eaten, allowing more room for the next food to enter your system. This is a very healthy, normal response and is the sign of a well-functioning digestive system.

With that said, having at least one bowel movement daily is good for your system. In order to achieve this, you must try to refrain from using laxatives. Constipation and bloating are major concerns and should be handled by a doctor. Find a functional medical doctor to address the issue of constipation. It's not a concern to be taken lightly.

Tip 10: Examine Your Stool

Don't be embarrassed. Take a closer look. Examine the quality of your stool. You should know the quality of its texture, smell, and size. Does it float above the water or sink to the bottom? You want to get to know your stool because any change in its color, shape, or weight can indicate a possible problem that needs to be addressed. If it doesn't appear to be normal, this may indicate an issue. Therefore, make sure you check your stool occasionally to look for any changes.

Conclusion

In brief, to help boost your digestive health for optimal activity, remove gluten-containing products from your diet, take probiotics and prebiotics, avoid sugar and prophylactic antibiotics, get tested for potential food allergies, take your time to chew food, check your stool quality, have a bowel movement at least once a day, consume fiber, and drink plenty of pure, filtered water.

In the following chapter, we'll discuss the gut-brain connection, which helps us to understand why medical treatments such as antidepressants and mind-body therapies like cognitive behavioral therapy are effective for IBS and other bowel-related disorders. Additionally, from a functional, more natural health standpoint, I personally know many people who have changed their diet and noticed a drastic difference in their mental health. Either way, science now understands that your gut is your second brain.

THE GUT-BRAIN CONNECTION

We are all familiar with the sayings: "a gut feeling," "anxiety felt at the pit of the stomach," "trust your gut instinct." These are not just idioms or phrases used metaphorically; there is a scientifically established connection between the gut and the brain!

The Enteric Nervous System (ENS)

There exists a second brain, a healing brain, a "saying" brain that serves as a link between our main brain and diseases. There exists a vast network of neurons that connect the brain and gut together. This network involves an array of chemicals and hormones that are continually sending signals regarding the environmental and internal factors that we are exposed to. This highly organized, intelligent expressway is called the brain-gut axis, and it is vigilant enough to constantly send signals about our internal functioning, any disharmony, our state of mind, etc. For example, remember a time you were anxious, and you experienced a queasy feeling in your stomach, or when you were excited, and you felt butterflies in your stomach? That is this network at work.

The brain and gut are intimately connected by the vagus nerve. The vagus nerve connects with most of the organs and plays a prominent role in activating the parasympathetic nervous system. Around 90% of the signals passing along the vagus nerve come not from the brain, but from the enteric (or intrinsic) nervous system to the brain. The brain and gut are intimately connected by the **vagus nerve**. The vagus nerve connects with most of the organs and plays a prominent role in activating the parasympathetic nervous system. Around 90 percent of the signals passing along the vagus nerve come not from the brain, but from the enteric nervous system to the brain.

THE FUNCTIONS OF THE ENTERIC NERVOUS SYSTEM

The enteric nervous system (ENS) is related to the autonomous nervous system (the parasympathetic and sympathetic that controls the involuntary mechanisms of our body like heart rate, respiration, and digestion). The ENS is composed of numerous neural circuits that oversee various motility functions, gut blood flow circulation, and mucosal transport secretions and its viscosity. The ENS looks over the immune and endocrine functions. The enteric neurons are contained in the myenteric plexus, which is a network of nerve fibers and ganglia between the longitudinal and circular muscle layers of the intestine. The submucous plexus is in the submucosal tissue, which connects the surface mucosal membrane lining to the deeper muscle layers in the stomach and intestines, which govern the neural circuits.

The gastrointestinal tract stands out amongst all the other organs of our body because of its interaction with various physicochemical stimuli from the outer environment in the form of ingested food. Hence, there needs to be a well-established harmony in the movements of its muscular apparatus so that there is optimum mixing and propulsion of the food during digestion, absorption, and excretion. This is achieved by the association of the neural apparatus with the muscular apparatus.

THE GUT ECOLOGY – OUR OWN INTERNAL ECOSYSTEM AND MICROBIOTA

Research has established the fact that our body is not only made up of millions of cells but also trillions of organisms that are called microbiome. The microbiome helps in the harmonious functioning of our internal systems. This microbiome is comprised of various types of symbiotic, commensal, and pathogenic bacteria (along with fungi and viruses) that inhabit our body and form our internal ecosystem. They are omnipresent in skin, genitals, oral cavity, eyes, and intestines. The bacteria residing in different regions are termed "microbiota." For example, gut microbiota are also referred to as "gut flora."

The gut microbiota plays an important role in digestion and the absorption of nutrients. Many gut microbiota exist in a symbiotic relationship with our body by providing us with much needed chemicals as a natural part of their metabolic cycle.

According to Georgetown University Hospital gastroenterologist Dr. Robynne Chutkan, "Any imbalance in this ecosystem gives rise to an array of health concerns ranging from certain types of cancer; autoimmune diseases like thyroid disorders, multiple sclerosis, and type 1 diabetes; as well as inflammatory bowel disease termed as Crohn's disease and irritable bowel syndrome."

The imbalance in the microbiome system can manifest as bloating, food intolerance, skin rashes, brain fog, and weight-loss resistance. The push for more antibacterial cleaning products and oral antibiotics endangers the vital microbiota that keep our internal ecosystem working for us and our body functioning well. I often encounter people who consume a probiotic as part of their daily regimen; however, it is important to note that one cannot completely counter the ill effects of antibiotics by only taking a probiotic. Hence, it is imperative to consume antibiotics only when absolutely necessary.

PROBIOTICS AND PREBIOTICS

Various drugs like steroids, hormones, acid blockers, and analgesics cause substantial harm to the microbiome, which affects the health of the intestinal mucosal lining and other organs. It is essential to replenish the lost flora so that the ecosystem is revived, but this cannot be done by simply taking a probiotic.

Diet is a crucial factor when it comes to rebuilding a healthy inner ecosystem and microbiome. As an example, food rich in prebiotics are onions, artichokes, lentils, leeks, oats, asparagus, and fermented foods that are rich in both prebiotics and probiotics like sauerkraut, kimchi, kefir, and pickles. Having a good balance of fermented foods can be very important in establishing a healthy microbiome; however, it is essential to first address any problems and imbalances in the microbiome before adding fermented foods.

Fecal microbiome transplant is an upcoming entity that has shown promising results in treating certain intestinal infections. Robynne Chutkan, MD, mentioned that it is also linked to treating certain autoimmune disorders, including irritable bowel syndrome, Crohn's disease, and ulcerative colitis. In fecal microbiota transplant, tested fecal material is placed in the patient via colonoscopy, endoscopy, sigmoidoscopy, or enema. It is done to replace the normal gut flora damaged by the use of antibiotics. It supposedly eradicates the bad bacteria, such as Clostridium difficile (C. diff.), that has overgrown as a result of antibiotics. C. diff. can cause severe, sometimes fatal, diarrhea. The CDC reports that 347,000 people in the U.S. alone were diagnosed with this infection in 2012.

AUTISM, GUT ECOLOGY, AND GLUTEN

Autism has a high prevalence rate of around 1 in 88 children. It is now well documented that autism spectrum disorders (ASDs) are affected by a disharmonious enteric ecosystem and that they are sensitive to the changes in the enteric microbiome.

In our post-industrial society, this disruption or disharmony in the enteric ecosystem can be multifactorial. It can be caused by a decline in exposure to symbiotic organisms; increased human migration; irrational, overuse of antibiotics, and changes in dietary habits. The metabolic and immune systems are sensitive to these changes in the enteric ecosystem and can cause changes in function and epigenetic expression. Autism, being a neurodevelopmental disorder, is highly sensitive to these changes if they occur during the periods of crucial brain development. This can also affect brain function in older children and adults as well. Such alterations may provoke or aggravate the formation of an ASD phenotype.

Gluten-derived peptides can trigger an immune response in children with ASD, and there is a possibility that these peptides could aggravate or trigger GI symptoms and behavioral concerns.

The research team at Penn State Medical concluded that a gluten-free diet aided in improving ASD behavior, physiological symptoms, and social behaviors in children suffering from GI distress in addition to allergy symptoms. There was also a noticeable enhancement with regard to children's social behavior, such as language, eye contact, engagement, attention span, behavior, and social responsiveness when a gluten-free diet was followed.

THE GUT AND ITS INFLUENCE ON MOODS AND FEELINGS

As previously established, there is a two-way communication between the brain and the gut microbiota known as the gut-brain axis. The gut microbiota, also called "the second brain," plays a vital role in influencing our mood. The symbiotic gut bacteria work on the hormonal level and help to reduce cortisol and adrenaline, both of which, in excessive amounts, are damaging to the body. Awareness of the connection of diet and mental health would lead to a reduction in many evitable psychological disorders. The gut microbiota plays a vital role in brain development, the evolution of our behavior, and reaction to stress, and it modifies the treatment for anxiety and depression. For ages, food has been known to play a major role in influencing our thoughts and moods. "Food is thy medicine" and "as is the food, so is the thought" are not just idioms; they are facts. We can shape our mental behavior and alter our mood through different foods. The following general guidelines and tips for a healthy eating plan will explore the gut and the important ways we can enhance its influence on our moods and feelings.

It's not just what we eat—it's how we eat. Incorporating mindfulness and awareness and staying in the moment while eating is as crucial as the type of food we eat. Mindless eating is associated with increased stress hormones and obesity.

What to Eat:

- fruits and vegetables, both raw and cooked, as they are loaded with nutrients and fiber
- herbs and spices, especially turmeric and saffron
- a handful of sprouted nuts and seeds daily
- foods that agree with your gut. Any food that causes bloating, gas, constipation, diarrhea, or reduced appetite should not be consumed.
- an appropriate amount of healthy fats, such as polyunsaturated fats that are high in omega-3s (linked to numerous health benefits, including that they affect parts of the brain associated with depression
- ample amounts of proteins
- probiotic foods, including kefir (unless dairy sensitive) and yogurt—ideally goat-milk yogurt, which is easier to digest and particularly high in probiotics like thermophilus, bifidus, and bulgaricus. Goat-milk yogurt can be infused with extra forms of probiotics like lactobacillus or acidophilus.
    - Kefir—a fermented dairy product and a blend of goat's milk and fermented kefir grains. It is high in lactobacilli and bifidus bacteria and antioxidants.

- Sauerkraut (fermented)—supplies probiotics that improve digestion. Microorganisms present in sauerkraut, including those of the lactobacillus bacteria genus, essentially "feed" the good bacteria in your gut, which improves digestive health. Sauerkraut also contains high levels of dietary fiber, as well as significant levels of vitamin A, vitamin C, vitamin K, and various B vitamins. It is a good source of iron, manganese, copper, sodium, magnesium, and calcium, in addition to contributing a moderate amount of protein to your diet.

- Dates and dark chocolate are very effective carriers of prebiotics. Dark chocolate helps to nourish the gut microbiome. Prebiotics are fibers in many plant-based foods we eat, and while we can't digest them, they pass through our colon where our beneficial microbes feast on them.

- Microalgae are superfoods from the ocean such as spirulina, chlorella, and blue-green algae. Microalgae acts as a prebiotic also in the way that it feeds and nourishes the probiotics present in your gut. These superfoods enhance the production of the beneficial bacteria and improve gastrointestinal health.

What Not to Eat:

- Being vigilant further helps us stay away from foods that could be toxic to both our gut and brain, such as being aware that processed food, especially deli and canned meat products, and food high in saturated fats, contributes to more dysbiosis or microbial imbalance in the gut. Avoid food high in refined sugars and gluten-rich food like wheat, barley, and rye (especially if sensitive to it).

How to Eat:

- Slowly and chew your food well.
- Only eat until you are satisfied, which is easier to sense when you eat slowly and chew well.
- Avoid any distraction while eating. Relax, CHEW, and enjoy your food.

WHAT ARE GMOS?

A GMO, or genetically modified organism, is a plant, animal, microorganism, or other organism whose genetic makeup has been modified in a laboratory using genetic engineering or transgenic technology. This technology creates combinations of plant, animal, bacterial, and viral genes that do not occur in nature or through traditional crossbreeding methods.

Most GMOs have been engineered to withstand the direct application of herbicides and/or to produce an insecticide. However, new technologies are being used to artificially develop other traits in plants, such as a resistance to browning in apples, and to create new organisms using synthetic biology. Despite biotech-industry promises, there is no evidence that any of the GMOs currently on the market offer increased yield, drought tolerance, enhanced nutrition, or any other consumer benefits.

Genetic modification affects many of the products we consume on a daily basis. The number of GMOs available for commercial use grows every year; however, the Non-GMO

Project works diligently to provide the most accurate, up-to-date standards for the non-GMO verification we see on packaging.

A growing body of evidence connects GMOs with health problems, environmental damage, and violation of farmers' and consumers' rights. More than 60 countries around the world, including Australia, Japan, and all the countries in the European Union, require GMOs to be labeled. Globally, there are 300 regions with outright bans on growing GMOs.

WHY ARE THEY CONSIDERED CONTROVERSIAL?

Scientifically speaking, there is no such thing as a "genetically modified organism" or GMO. Genetic modification is a process, not a final product. GMO has become widely embraced as a shorthand way to refer to a plant or animal with new traits that have been created through modern genetic manipulation, often through transgenesis. In this process, genetic material (DNA) from unrelated species is combined synthetically and/or heavily modified and inserted into the organism's genetic code. But developing an all-encompassing, scientifically accurate definition of this highly politicized term is difficult, if not impossible, which poses challenges for regulators.

For centuries, farmers have used breeding to modify the genetics of plans, searching for ways to improve traits that include a healthier yield, resist disease, and improve flavor. Some of those breeding techniques, including wide cross-breeding and mutagenizing seeds using radiation or chemicals, involved years of laboratory tinkering, but still are not considered GMOs as the term is commonly used. Mutation breeding exposes *seeds* to chemicals or radiation to generate mutants with desirable traits to be bred with other cultivars. Advancements in biotechnology over recent decades have given breeders the ability to exert greater and more precise control over the breeding process. Today, the seeds genetically engineered by companies represent the majority of what is planted in U.S. farmlands, particularly in grain crops. The foods that result from them are popularly referred to as GMOs.

The subject of genetically modified organisms is one of the most highly debated food and environmental topics in the world today. Just look at the response to Chipolte's recent announcement that the chain would cease including GMO ingredients on its menu. Health advocates applauded the move as a step in the right direction on the heels of Whole Foods' 2013 commitment to label all GMO products in its stores by 2018. Detractors called it yet another example of a hypocritical food maker using unsubstantiated claims to sell food, given that the chain will continue to serve soda, which contains high-fructose corn syrup made with genetically modified corn.

At the crux of the controversy are a number of unknowns about the long-term health effects of ingesting genetically modified foods and the impact these plans and accompanying farming methods have on the environment. With some experts saying that in recent years, 60 to 70 percent of food products will contain GMOs, it's clear that to advance this issue is central to the future of our food supply. To answer some commonly asked questions and encourage a constructive dialogue on the topic, the following offers a brief overview of the facts that stand today.

WHAT ACTUALLY HAPPENS TO FOOD THAT HAS BEEN GENETICALLY MODIFIED?

In a genetic modification (or engineering) of food, scientists remove one or more genes from the DNA of another organism, such as a bacterium, virus, animal or plant, and recombine them into the DNA of the plant they want to alter. By adding these new genes, genetic engineers hope the plant will express the traits associated with the genes. For example, genetic engineers have transferred genes from a bacterium known as Bacillus thuringiensis, or Bt, into the DNA of corn. Bt is a toxin that kills insects by breaking open their stomachs. Even though we were told that only insects would be affected by the Bt toxin, it has been shown to harm some of the cells of the human digestive system.

One of the main problems with genetic engineering is that the process of inserting genes into the DNA of a food plant is quite random; scientists have no idea where the genes will go. This can disrupt the functioning of other genes and create novel proteins that have never been in our food supply before, and potentially create food that can be toxic to us, thereby increasing food intolerances and allergies.

GM foods are developed–and marketed–because there is some perceived advantage to either the producer or consumer of these foods. This is meant to translate into a product with a lower price, greater benefit in terms of durability or nutritional value, or both. Initially, GM seed developers wanted their products to be accepted by producers and have concentrated innovations that bring direct benefit to farmers and the food industry in general.

One of the objectives for developing plants based on GMOs is to improve crop protection. The GM crops currently on the market are mainly aimed at an increased level of crop protection through the introduction of resistance against plant diseases caused by insects or viruses, or through increased tolerance toward herbicides.

HOW DOES THE BODY PERCEIVE GENETICALLY MODIFIED FOOD?

Genetically modified foods (GMFs) have been on the market for some time and make up a significant portion of the food most people eat. How aware is the general population of the prevalence of genetically modified foods in their diet? There is reason to believe that the level of awareness regarding GMFs and the understanding of the technology behind GMFs is not vast.

You do not have to look hard to find genetically modified food on supermarket shelves: More than 85 percent of the corn and soy grown in the United States comes from seeds whose DNA has been genetically modified to increase yields. These two crops play starring roles in countless processed foods, from soda to salad dressing to bread. Advocates say genetically modified (GM) foods enable farmers to produce more with fewer chemicals, which means a cleaner environment and cheaper groceries for us all. But the question remains: what impact do GM foods have on our health?

The answer is that no-one really knows. GM foods have been on the market only since 1994, and research on their long-term effects on humans is scarce. To date, most of the studies have been done on animals; worryingly, though, some of those studies link GM foods to altered metabolism, inflammation, kidney and liver malfunction, and reduced fertility. In one experiment, multiple generations of hamsters were fed a diet of GM soy; by the third generation, they were losing the ability to produce offspring, producing about half as many pups as the non-GM soy group.

In addition, allergy sufferers worry that, as genes are transferred among plants, allergenic proteins (from peanuts or wheat) will pop up in unexpected places (like soy or sugar). Richard Goodman, PhD, a professor of food science and technology at the University of Nebraska-Lincoln and a former scientist for Monsanto, says that seed companies run sophisticated tests to prevent that kind of mistake from happening. But inserting new genes into a seed's delicately constructed genome is always a gamble because scientists cannot predict all the consequences.

WHAT IS THE CONNECTION BETWEEN GMOS AND DISEASE?

Because the body does not recognize this foreign GMO food, it cannot fully break it down and assimilate it properly. These food proteins that are not digested fully can, over time, escape into the bloodstream, causing your body's immune system to go on high alert, producing an inflammatory response. This can happen slowly or quickly as a person becomes allergic to the proteins in food that escaped into their bloodstream. The obesity epidemic and the inflammatory epidemic are directly connected, and until people start consuming natural, non-GMO foods, there will be health issues related to weight gain, allergic reactions, indigestion, pain, etc. Of course, limiting the obvious other offending foods such as transfats, sugars, and caffeine will help decrease weight issues, inflammation, and pain as well.

Inflammation and Autoimmune Conditions

Many people are unaware that they are consuming foods derived from genetically modified organisms. If they suffer from inflammation of their intestinal tract and don't know how to eliminate the foods that are causing it, the result will be a hyperpermeability of the intestinal lining, or as previously noted, leaky gut.

GMOs have been associated with autoimmune conditions and such conditions as autism, diabetes, Parkinson's disease, Graves' disease, and Hashimoto's Thyroiditis. The thyroid is an endocrine organ that secretes the thyroid hormone. Thyroid dysfunction has been identified with mood disorders. Depression is frequently associated with low levels of thyroid hormone (hypothyroidism), while mood elevation is often associated with high levels of thyroid hormone (hyperthyroidism). Endocrine-disrupting chemicals (EDC) that cause erratic behavior have been linked, e.g., between food additives and neurotoxicity in cells and hyperactive behavior in children. Incidents have been reported of laboratory rats and farm animals exhibiting uncharacteristic aggressive and antisocial behavior when being fed a diet consisting of GMO soy or corn. There are further risks associated with eating unfermented soy if a person has a thyroid dysfunction, and studies have shown there is a link between thyroid disruption and neurological diseases. Thyroid hormones are critical to the development of the fetal and neonatal brain, as well as to many other aspects of pregnancy and fetal growth.

Obesity

Another topic is obesity. First, let's start with the definition of obesity. According to the Endocrine Society, "Obesity occurs when, over time, the body takes in more calories than it burns."

When a person's body mass index (BMI) is over 30, that person is considered obese.

Because obesity is related to the number of calories a person consumes, a GM crop would have to contain considerably more calories than non-GM varieties of that crop to be linked to obesity. But the fact is that GM crops are carefully reviewed to make sure they are substantially equivalent to non-GM crops in their composition and nutritional qualities. This includes levels of protein, carbohydrate, fat, vitamin, mineral, fiber, and moisture, among others. The caloric value of food from a GM plant will be in the same range as that of the comparable non-GM plant. There is, however, concern regarding high fructose corn syrup (HFDS), which is made primarily from GM corn, which may be one of the biggest culprits contributing to the rise in obesity.

Whatever is causing obesity today, it isn't the calories from GM plants. Some people have claimed that GM crops cause obesity in ways unrelated to the caloric content of the food. However, more than 150 studies have been conducted, and the results of these studies do not provide any cause for concern about weight gain or other negative impacts from GMOs. That said, excessive caloric intake, regardless of the source, combined with inadequate physical activity, are the primary causes of obesity.

Some companies are using genetic modification to improve the nutritional value of crops, such as soybeans. These nutritionally "improved" GM soybeans contain more oleic acid—an unsaturated fatty acid found in olive oil—and significantly fewer saturated fatty acids than traditional soybeans.

ADD/ADHD

The increase in ADD/ADHD is yet another concern related to GMOs. Before we get into potential causes for the increase in its prevalence, let›s define ADD/ADHD. ADD, or attention deficit disorder, has largely been replaced with ADHD or Attention Deficit Hyperactivity Disorder. involve a cluster of symptoms that include inattention, hyperactivity, and impulsive behaviors. Children with ADHA often struggle in school and have difficulty managing interpersonal relationships. They also tend to suffer from lower self-esteem.

Diagnosing ADHD comes down to a matter of opinion, as there is no physical test, like a brain scan, that can pinpoint the condition. This could change. According to a recent study a newer MRI method called magnetic field correlation imaging detects low iron levels in the brains of children with ADHD, which could potentially help parents and patients to make better-informed decisions about treatment.

Another important point is that children's bodies develop at a fast pace and are more likely to be influenced by and show the effects of GM foods. That is why independent scientists used adolescent rats in their FM feeding studies. The rats showed significant health damage after only 10 days, including damaged immune systems and digestive function; smaller brains, livers and testicles; partial atrophy of the liver; and potentially precancerous cell growth in the intestines.

WHAT CAN WE DO?

I have always encouraged eating clean foods that are organic. One reason is to avoid the xenohormones fed to livestock, as well as the pesticides and herbicides sprayed on produce. Another reason is to avoid GMOs.

The primary genetically modified foods include corn, soy, canola oil, and cottonseed oil. If you don't eat a 100 percent organic diet, at the very least you want to avoid these foods and oils. Many people reading this already try to avoid unfermented soy, but some aren't aware of the health issues with genetically modified corn. Therefore, if you buy anything that has corn in it, make sure it is either organic or is labeled as a non-GMO on the packaging.

We also need to be thorough when reading ingredients, as its stands to reason that cornmeal, corn syrup, and cornstarch are all derived from corn. However, other ingredients may not be as obvious, such as caramel and baking power (from cornstarch), and ascorbic acid is made from corn syrup (yet another reason to consume high-quality vitamin C complex that has high bioavailability).

Today, the use of GM crops is widely debated. GM foods available on the international market have passed risk assessments and are not likely to present risks for human health. In addition, no effects have been shown on human health by the general population in the countries where they have been approved.

As with gluten and other things we ingest, we need to be in charge of and vigilant with our choices, as much as possible.

THREE THEORIES OF EATING

No. 1: The thrifty genotype

This theory discusses the process of evolution and how it has given an advantage to humans who are genetically predisposed to have a strong appetite and the capability of depositing excess calories in the form of body fat for survival purposes. If we stored energy in the form of fat, based on this theory, we could survive longer, even during periods when food was scarce.

No. 2: The sugar/fatty-acid cycle

This theory studies the actual mechanism that free fatty acids from our fat deposits and our blood sugar antagonize each other to be used as a fuel source for various bodily functions. This is a complex theory to comprehend, but the logic behind it this: if you burn fatty acids as your main fuel source (this happens during periods of fasting), you will be able to reduce the necessity of protein metabolization, sparing any muscle tissue from being used as an energy source. Thus, burning body fat as fuel during periods of fasting enables you to maintain all your muscle mass because your body is getting its energy from mobilizing fatty acids and glucose. Therefore, contrary to what many believe, you will not lose muscle mass when fasting.

No 3: Feast-and-famine cycle

This theory was based on the fact that everything in nature occurs in cycles, and it focuses on the connection between insulin and growth hormone (GH). This theory illustrates how we can utilize calories from the foods that we eat and at the same time burn unwanted body fat from our bodies without sacrificing our muscle mass.

These three concepts, initially formed in the 1960s, were revolutionary and sparked much controversy, which we still encounter today. The next thing we will explore is fasting as a pattern-of-eating approach. Fasting is still a confusing, controversial diet topic, yet these three eating theories have managed to set the foreground for fasting studies, evaluations, and further development.

THE WONDERFUL BENEFITS OF INTERMITTENT FASTING

Often called an eating pattern, intermittent fasting (IF) is a term used to describe a way of eating that alternates between periods of fasting and periods of eating food regularly. This is a very powerful tool that I started practicing when I was 20 years old. When done correctly, it's not only a great way to significantly bring down markers of inflammation, but it also offers many other amazing health benefits. Fasting enables the system to take a break from depositing fat and to use it instead for energy!

There is good logic behind this way of eating. Humans have been fasting ever since we have been in existence, simply because food was scarce in certain periods, especially during long, cold winters, and in some nations and religions (such as Christianity and Islam), fasting became the norm.

Culturally, we are wired to consume our food at certain times of the day: breakfast at nine, lunch at one, and dinner at eight, for example. The truth of the matter is a lot of controversy surrounds the subject of eating and when we should consume certain meals to facilitate weight loss and good health and when we should not.

Consider these benefits of fasting:

- reduced body fat
- reduced blood-sugar levels
- reduced amounts of insulin and insulin resistance
- accelerated fat burning and fat oxidation
- raised levels of growth hormone
- reduced levels of cortisol
- reduced digestive stress
- reduced chronic inflammation

These are some amazing health benefits, so let's take a closer look at how fasting helps and affects our bodies in six different ways:

No. 1: Reduces insulin

Insulin is the primary hormone that tells your body whether to store energy or burn it. When you eat, your insulin level goes up, and the higher levels of insulin signal your body to store energy. When you are not eating, insulin falls, telling your body to release energy. Therefore, people with insulin resistance have a harder time losing weight because their body is in a constant high-insulin state and they are always storing fat. Working away just behind your stomach region is another organ called the pancreas, which produces the insulin. Blood-glucose levels and other hormonal compounds control the release of insulin. In a healthy person, insulin creation and circulation are strongly controlled procedures that enable the body to stabilize its metabolic requirements. Insulin is the main compound that sends the message to your body and brain to deposit energy from food and to activate the storage mode.

When you eat, regardless of whether it is healthy or unhealthy food, insulin levels start to rise. This is one reason that eating regularly (multiple meals per day) can lead to a sustained spike of insulin levels and all the symptoms that may possibly come with insulin resistance, such as inflammation, diabetes, heart issues, and even certain types of cancer.

So, what does insulin have to do with fasting? Insulin levels drop when you fast, which is favorable for fighting inflammation and triggering fat loss, among other health benefits.

No. 2: Controls blood sugar

Blood sugar (glucose) is the level of sugar found in our blood. When we consume excessive amounts of food (mainly carbohydrates and sugar), our pancreas goes on overload and begins spitting out loads of insulin as it tries to catch up with the sudden rise and supply of sugar in our bloodstream.

Even periods of short fasting (12 hours) enable our body to control blood glucose, but the question is raised about its benefit for people with hypoglycemia.

Diagnosing the "low sugar" or "hypoglycemia" condition is accomplished best by symptoms alone, opposed to a specific blood glucose number. After testing hundreds of patients' fasting blood-glucose levels, I have learned that hypoglycemia is not diagnosed by a test alone. Some people (including myself) that I have tested who are working on keeping their carbohydrate intake low will show 40 to 50 mg/dl (which is still within the physiological range) at night or during periods of no food, and yet they will have zero hypoglycemic symptoms. However, for someone who is hypoglycemic or is used to having their blood sugars at 170 to 190, dropping suddenly to 40 to 50 could put them at serious risk.

While I believe 80 percent of the population would likely benefit from water fasting, there are several definite contraindications. If any of the following apply to you, you should NOT do any extended types of fasting:

- Malnourished or underweight (having a body mass index (BMI) of 18.5 or less)
- Individuals with severe eating disorders including anorexia nervosa and bulimia nervosa. (Even though I was well read on the topic of fasting, I didn't seek the help of a trained physician and therefore fasted inappropriately, subsequently causing more harm to my health without realizing it until later.)
- Children should not fast longer than 24 hours because their bodies need nutrients for growth and development. If your child needs to lose weight, a much safer approach is eliminating all refined grains and sugars.
- Pregnant and/or breastfeeding women need a steady supply of nutrients for their baby's healthy growth and development. Fasting is simply too risky.
- If you are on certain medications like metformin, aspirin, and any other drug that might cause stomach upset or ulcers or, if you are on any diabetic medications, this is especially risky and should be avoided at all costs.

No. 3: Stimulates fat burning

The process of fat burning is called "lipolysis" in scientific terms. During this phase, fatty acids are freed and circulate throughout the bloodstream to be used as energy sources by your muscle tissue and vital organs.

Based on the latest research, your body is able to burn higher amounts of fat in four to eight hours since the last time you ate something, and the effects begin to slow after 30 hours. If you fast between 12 and 14 hours, you will start triggering fat burning as your main energy source. Given these facts, there is no need to fast for longer periods of time.

No. 4: Raises growth hormone (GH) levels

Fasting stimulates growth hormone release. When you combine this with exercise and healthy sleep patterns, it is the perfect combination for achieving healthy weight loss and loads of mental clarity and energy. GH is at its peak during your teenage years (this probably explains why during our teenage years we eat our parents out of house and home). The wonderful thing about growth hormone is that it helps enhance muscle volume. Fasting has been demonstrated to raise growth hormone levels, which dispels the myth that fasting leads to muscle loss. If you pair this with a solid workout regimen and good sleep, you will have a full-blown muscle-building program that gets you the results you are looking for.

No. 5: Reduces inflammation

Our systems respond to inflammation through a process named "acute inflammatory response," which is triggered by damaged or injured tissue, which is when inflammation at its essence is a good thing. It protects us and works to eliminate the cause of the damage (e.g., bee sting, scraped knee, etc.).

Some of the most frequent inflammatory diseases people suffer with today are diabetes, heart problems, low-grade infections, autoimmune conditions (such as rheumatoid arthritis and Hashimoto's thyroiditis), asthma, and, of course, even normal everyday aging.

No. 6: Triggers rejuvenation and cleansing on a cellular level

When I refer to IF, I am not referring to just any old master cleansing or detoxification program. I am referring to *autophagy*, a physiological process that takes place in the body and that handles cell organelle damage. Fasting can support autophagy.

Why do we need autophagy? The process of cleansing our cells of debris has caught the attention of cancer researchers who see it as a potential treatment for cancer, as well as Alzheimer's and Parkinson's diseases. Researchers have shown that fasting just twice a week could reduce the risk of developing Alzheimer's and Parkinson's diseases.

Healthy dietary habits, as well as positive changes in exercise and sleep patterns, have been found to strongly impact brain function in a positive way. Children suffering from epileptic episodes experience them far less when fasting or following calorie-restriction diets. It is estimated that fasting helps trigger protective functions that help control the overstimulated brain signals of epileptic patients. Some children have also shown some improvement from following a higher-fat, lower-carbohydrate diet (e.g., ketogenic diet).

However, it is not just the brains of epileptics who experience overstimulation. Given all the bits of information coming in at any point of the day, we all suffer from this overstimulation in our everyday lives. Those of us with supposed "normal" brain function experience another form of imbalance and overexcitement, which affects brain focus and function. This is especially true when we are being overfed, as supported by Dr. Mattson and fellow researcher in relevant studies published in the journal *Nature Reviews Neuroscience*.

Another study conducted by University of California researchers demonstrated that periods of fasting can protect against the destruction of the immune system and even accelerate its recovery. They found that fasting changes cells from an idle status to a status of self-rejuvenation. Fasting essentially stimulated cellular regeneration in an organ or tissue.

In clinical studies carried out in human subjects who were going through chemotherapy, the patients did not eat for prolonged periods of time. This resulted in lower levels of white blood cells circulating in the blood. In studies with mice, periods of fasting switched on a regenerative process, altering the communication pathways for blood-building and immune-boosting stem cells.

Simply, fasting triggers the death of already damaged and weak immunity cells, so that when the system goes through such a transitional backup stage, it produces healthier new cells.

A collection of numerous scientific studies on the subject of fasting was featured in the *American Journal of Nutrition.* The study overview considered many human and animal studies and concluded that fasting can be a useful preventive measure for heart disease, cancer, and diabetes because it lowers the risk of developing such diseases.

A study at the University of Utah found that individuals who fasted for even one day per month had 40 percent less risk of experiencing arterial plaquing as opposed to those who did not fast.

Some of the concerns my patients have:

- How can I make fasting fit into my schedule?
- Will it be an easy process to implement?
- What are the typical mistakes people make, and how can they be avoided?
- How will I feel?
- Will it be difficult? How will my day go?
- Will I lead a normal life or go through another failed diet attempt?

First, you must realize that intermittent fasting (IF) is not just another "diet." What makes it different from a "diet" is described below.

Adherence and Consistency

Adherence is a vital component of, or should we say *trigger* for, success when following a new way of eating or workout plan. It is adherence paired with consistency that makes our attempts successful.

As a matter of fact, if we are trying to maintain a way of eating that is too strict and hard to follow, chances are we will struggle to follow through and abandon it before we see any long-term results.

ADOPTING A NEW WAY OF LIVING

A study conducted in 2010 with 390 human subjects (featured in *Appetite*) reveals that a diet's complexity correlates with the level of adherence. The researchers found that the more complex a way of eating was to follow, the higher the risk people would quit their mentally demanding weight-loss plan. Conversely, the easier the way of eating and the fewer restrictions it had, the more likely people would follow it, stick to it for longer, and finally succeed in their attempt to lose weight.

Similar findings were also observed in the study of Jutta Matta and her group of researchers at the Max Planck Institute for Human Development, which studies human development through interdisciplinary projects. Their study was also featured in *Appetite* (2007). The researchers studied over 1,200 subjects (a very impressive number) who followed various diets. They studied popular weight-loss diet types with very strict, excessive rules and concluded that diets with stricter rules/demands are linked with lower levels of adherence by the subjects. They also added that perceived difficulty (how difficult the person thought the diet was) is an indicator that they will give up prematurely, before their initial milestone and before seeing any results.

After many years of witnessing patients follow specific "diets" or ways of eating, I realized that in many of our short-term diet programs, our patients follow them perfectly for about four to six weeks, all while they are also offered plenty of guidance, support, and motivation to stick to it. Once the plan finishes, however, they quickly switch back to their former ways.

Even though our body's nutritional demands and physiological makeup are complicated, our ways of eating do not have to be. This is why intermittent fasting is so beneficial. It is not just another diet requiring you to eat this and that; it is simply an eating pattern. You still want to choose whole, healthy foods that are not loaded with refined sugar and grains, but this eating pattern is easier to adopt into your life than any "diet."

So how can you be most successful in this lifestyle change? What makes IF different from other diets?

1. IF requires that you do not eat for arranged periods of time and drink plenty of plain liquids like water, water with a splash of apple cider vinegar, and/or black coffee or tea during your fasting time.
2. IF enables you to save some cash. Perhaps you have already begun using that "protein shake" or "juicing protocol detox" diet only to be floored by the exorbitant prices of supplements and foods you must take in. Do not get me wrong—specific supplementation can be necessary, depending on your current state of health, but without guidance this can be more expensive than necessary. It is also difficult to stick

with something like this for long periods of time. I've found that many people are not willing to take handfuls of pill-form supplements or drink protein and juiced liquids for meals for long periods of time. On the contrary, the cost of fasting is zero to none. There is no need to buy supplements, ready-made meals, or the like.

3. IF improves your productivity. Many people tell us that once they try intermittent fasting, they feel more energetic and rejuvenated. Thus, they can carry out daily tasks in a more productive way. Your brain will play tricks on you, sending you the signal that you need to eat. You can control this with a bit of practice and patience. Another benefit is that you will save time meal prepping.
4. IF enables you to develop a new bond with food (believe it or not, this can happen). Most of our patients are assisted in some way with their eating issues. Some of them are undereating, some are eating huge amounts of food, while others engage in binge eating, depending on their mood. The bottom line is relationships with food have become very complex, and having a practitioner trained to help you sort through this can be very helpful.
5. IF helps us develop new sustainable habits. I want to be honest with you—you are probably going to feel a bit hungry once you start intermittent fasting. Your system is accustomed to eating regularly and usually every few hours. For example, when you wake up, it is natural to feel hungry. A study conducted in 2006 found that almost half our daily actions (around 40 percent) were not from intrinsic decisions,

but from learned or familiar habits. The study has shown that when someone starts to form a new habit, like hitting the gym twice a week for example, it can become automatic over time. Other studies have noticed that most families do not have plans to eat fast food regularly. What typically happens, though, is that habit of having fast food once or twice a month easily becomes once a week or more, which leads to eating unhealthy junk food more often without realizing it. Fasting, as in the case of other habits, requires time, practice, and patience until it also becomes automatic. By developing the pattern of intermittent fasting, we allow space for new healthy habits to form.

6. IF has options. There is no single way to implement it. For example, some people suggest taking six meals per day, but that eating pattern may be challenging and make you feel unable to keep it up. We are all busy with life, so that way of eating may not be so easy for you. Since there are numerous different fasting patterns, it is important that you adopt one that is suitable for you and your lifestyle. Meticulously planning your regimen paves the way to achieving any goals. We recommend that you consult with one of our physicians or a holistic nutrition coach (or someone else who understands this process) to help you develop a personalized intermittent fasting plan. Our practice offers multiple plans, resources, and referrals in our area that can help.

To put it simply, many of our patients have stated that intermittent fasting has improved their connection with food. Once we bring intermittent fasting into practice, food no longer controls us, and once you are ready to eat, you are going to enjoy every bite. You will save time and energy, and you will enjoy your food. IF helps put you in the driver's seat when it comes to eating. You will be the one in charge of your relationship with food, and your food choices will be enjoyable and guilt-free.

TYPICAL QUESTIONS/CONCERNS ABOUT IF

No. 1: What about breakfast? Currently, there are no solid scientific data deeming breakfast is just as important as lunch and dinner. However, to our patients with symptoms of hypoglycemia (hangry, nauseous, low energy, sugar cravings, difficulty losing weight, etc.), I always recommend eating something in the morning, even if it is just a small bite of something with quality protein to help stabilize blood sugars at the start of the day. There is also evidence that while people who do eat breakfast might do a bit better in weight-loss diets, it is not breakfast itself that triggers this fat loss but their increased exercise and better food choices. If you are a breakfast lover and would rather not skip, that is perfectly fine. There are other options you can choose to adjust your schedule. For example, you can take your breakfast choices at another time of the day or follow an IF program that includes one main meal in the morning, i.e., breakfast.

No. 2: What happens with starvation mode? There is this widespread notion that when you restrict your calories excessively, even for temporary periods of time, you will cease to lose body fat because your metabolism switches to a process called "starvation mode" and your metabolic speed slows down. Although many weight-loss plans and products support this notion, the physiology is not correct.

Our metabolic functions rely heavily on energetic expenditures necessary to keep our cells alive, but the food we eat is not as closely connected to our metabolism as we may think. Therefore, IF doesn't negatively affect our metabolic function. Our metabolism has a major connection to our lean body mass, however, which implies that if you aren't following a strengthening workout, you should be!

No. 3: What if I am hungry? This is normal at the very beginning, but as we discussed previously, switching eating patterns is not an overnight process. You will need plenty of time, patience, and practice to make it a natural part of your lifestyle. We further suggest that you consult an IF coach for additional guidance and support. It can make a world of a difference. During the first few days of IF, you may feel hungry during the hours you used to eat. After all, you may have followed the same eating pattern for years (e.g., eating breakfast in the morning), so change is not easy. The initial days of IF may feel uncomfortable, as has been reported, but if you are patient enough, your system will become accustomed and IF will become a wonderful, health-promoting habit.

IF PLANS

- **EAT-STOP-EAT** (fast for 24 hours once or twice a week)

It is hard to talk about 24-hour fasting windows without giving credit to Brad Pilon and his book *Eat Stop Eat*, a great resource on the topic of If. The regimen calls for one to two 24-hour fasting periods per week on days that suit your daily schedule (like the weekend, perhaps). Pilon writes that it is possible to be healthy, energetic, and lean without paying too much attention to your food choices. We can achieve this by being the kind of individual who notices, since we do not need to eat all the time, that what we choose to eat is up to us, and by also acknowledging the value of physical workouts. However, I personally believe that we should pay attention to our food choices, whether using IF or not, as this will take us to greater levels of health the fastest way possible.

- **5:2 Diet:** (five days of typical eating and two days of clean eating)

The 5:2 IF pattern calls for eating as usual for five days in a week and fasting for the remaining two days of the week (taking in only 500 calories). The protocol considers the evidence of IF paired with an eating plan that is low in calories to allow weight loss without starvation. This plan offers a very nutritionally stabilized intake (founded on a Mediterranean style of diet), and it easily becomes a part of most schedules as it lets you choose the two days you are going to fast/eat fewer calories.

For example, there was one study with 100 female subjects split into two groups. One group consumed 25 percent fewer calories every day, while the other group was following the 5:2 fasting pattern, fasting for only two days of the week. While both groups eventually lost weight after a period of six months following these plans, the group following the 5:2 diet lost more belly fat and showed more balanced blood-sugar levels on blood tests.

- **16:8 IF plan:** (16 hours of fasting and eight hours of eating normally)

Also called "the leangains method," this is my personal choice when it comes to IF, and it is probably the most popular. Martin Berkhan, a nutritional consultant, writer, and personal trainer, made this IF method famous by initiating the "lean-gains" act, which encourages a 16-hour fasting window, followed by eight hours of normal eating. This is a highly versatile IF plan, and again, you can choose which 16 hours you will be fasting, and which eight hours you will be eating normally. Most people choose sleeping hours to cover a portion of their sixteen-hour fasting period and eat normally between 11 a.m. and 7 p.m.

- **Warrior Mode:** (24 hours of fasting and four hours of eating)

  The warrior mode calls for fasting for 20 consecutive hours and eating only for four, usually at dinnertime, but the four-hour window can be moved around. All the calories you will need for the day will be taken during that time. Many people who have adopted this method use the 3 p.m. to 7 p.m. dinnertime period. This is one of the most aggressive IF methods, and many of those that tried this reported saving huge amounts of valuable time. You only need to prep one meal per day, with no snacks or anything else "eating" your time. All your daily calories will be taken during this single meal, so you can get a longer fasting window.

In the next chapter, we will discuss the difference between genetics and epigenetics, as well as how our environment can alter our genetic expression of certain genes. Epigenetics explains why a line of family members can all carry genes for a type of cancer; however, altering the lifestyle and dietary choices of individuals in that same family can essentially keep cancer genes from expressing. The science shows that we can live our lives free from the worry and fear that we may also develop cancer or a heart attack like Dad and Grandpa did. What an empowering thought!

GENETICS VS. EPIGENETICS

Genetics and epigenetics are areas of science that have always fascinated me. We have the genes for certain characteristics, personality traits, and illnesses, yet our environment has everything to do with the expression of certain genes being turned on or off. That astounds me.

Genetics is an area of science concerned with the study of genes, heredity, and genetic variation in living organisms. The father of genetics is Gregor Mendel. He studied and described the mechanism of trait-inheritance patterns where different traits of an organism are passed from the parent organism to the offspring. He said that such inheritance occurred through the passing of a particular unit of inheritance from one generation to the next. Mendel used garden pea plants to explain these phenomena. In the modern world, the unit of inheritance is referred to as a gene.

Genes are present in an organism's chromosomes, which are composed of both DNA and protein. In the past, scientists could not differentiate the molecule of inheritance between DNA and protein present in the chromosome. But more recently, given different scientific experiments, it was confirmed that the DNA is the molecule responsible for inheritance. Therefore, genetic information to be passed from one generation to the next is stored within the molecules of DNA.

Epigenetics is the study of heritable changes in gene expression (active versus inactive genes) that do not involve changes to the underlying DNA sequence—a change in phenotype without a change in genotype—which in turn affects how cells read the genes. Epigenetics means that your body can turn certain genes on and off. This means that through epigenetics, you can literally change your genetic makeup depending on internal and external environmental factors such as diet and lifestyle.

The epigenetic change is a regular, natural occurrence that can also be influenced by several factors including age, the environment, lifestyle, and disease state. Epigenetic modifications can manifest as commonly as the manner in which cells terminally differentiate to end up as skin cells, liver cells, brain cells, etc.

Epigenetics is the alteration in heritable traits in gene expression that does not involve changes to the DNA sequence. In other words, it is the change in the phenotype (the set of observable characteristics of an individual resulting from the interaction of its genotype with the environment) without changing the genotype (the genetic constitution of an individual organism). Repressor proteins, which are attached to the silencer regions of the DNA, control gene expression. Epigenetics takes place naturally and regularly, but it can be caused by the external and internal environment of someone's body, age, and disease conditions.

For example, newborn rats were picked up and petted for three minutes every day for a few weeks. As adults, these rats had lower levels of stress hormones, better learning and memory, and were more neurologically intact when reaching old age than a non-petted counterpart.

Simply put, you can turn certain genes off and on depending on the stimuli that you provide your body. Genes can change due to the demands of the environment. When we are born, our bodies do not know what type of environment into which we are being born. Therefore, we have a built-in change mechanism that can be activated and shaped by the external environment.

It is not fully understood how this works, but it is an extremely exciting discovery that further reinforces the autonomy that we have over our lives and circumstances.

HOW DOES ENVIRONMENT AFFECT GENES?

The expression of genes in an organism can be influenced by the environment, including the external world in which the organism is located or develops, as well as the organism's internal world, which includes such factors as its hormones and metabolism. One major internal environmental influence that affects gene expression is gender, as is the case with sex-influenced and sex-limited traits. Similarly, drugs, chemicals, temperature, and light are among the external environmental factors that can determine which genes are turned on and off, thereby influencing the way an organism develops and functions.

When the first human genome was decoded, the popular thinking went: "If we know the genes, we know the person." Today, almost 15 years later, science is in the middle of an exciting new area of research. The field alleges that traumatic experiences can be passed down through the generations and even significantly affect the lives of grandchildren. As it turns out, the reality is that genes not only control, but are also controlled. And that is what epigenetics is all about—how genes are controlled and what factors can influence them?

Epigenetic refers to the meta level of genetic regulation. Under the influence of external factors, epigenetic mechanisms regulate which genes are turned on and off. This helps our fixed genetic material to be more flexible. At the microbiochemical level, epigenetic regulators are responsible for how closely packed individual genomic regions are and, therefore, how accessible or not they are. This works by small adhered or detached chemical groups. The resulting marking of the genome is read by specialized enzymes that then cause the switching on or off of the genes.

While the sequence of DNA may not be affected by your environment, the way genes work (called gene expression) can. Think of DNA as a computer's hardware; there may be several types of software programs that can regulate what the hardware does. Epigenetics is the study of heritable changes in gene expression that don't involve changing the underlying DNA—effectively, software changes that alter gene function.

Environmental factors such as food, drugs, or exposure to toxins can cause epigenetic changes by altering the way molecules bind to DNA or by changing the structure of proteins that DNA wraps around. These structural changes can result in slight changes in gene activity; they can also produce more dramatic changes by switching genes on when they should be off or vice versa.

HOW GENES AFFECT THE HEALTH OF CHILDREN?

Genes affect your chances of having several common or uncommon illnesses, such as heart disease, asthma, and diabetes, but so do many other factors, such as diet and lifestyle. As we talked about earlier, when diet and lifestyle are changed for the better, you change the way your genes express themselves; therefore, you have better health outcomes. It is like betting on a horse race—the horse, rider, course, and weather can all affect the outcome in a way that is hard to predict.

Studies confirm that most aspects of human growth and development are strongly influenced by the genetic makeup of the child. For instance, comparing identical and nonidentical twins shows large genetic components for such physical differences as height and weight, as well as for many behaviors, including learning ability. One example of this is parents carrying the genetic defect called MTHFR (or 5,10-methylenetetrahydrofolate reductase). The MTHFR gene defect can affect your body's ability to methylate (detoxify). There is an association with MTHFR and midline defects like tongue-tie (a short frenulum that restricts tongue movement) that can drastically affect the breastfeeding relationship between mother and child. This is a common occurrence that I see in most of my new infant patients presenting to my office.

There are four types of "ties," depending on placement in the mouth. These ties can affect breastfeeding in infancy, as well as speech and development of the mouth and teeth as the child ages. Other midline defects that are associated with MTHRF are lip-tie, sacral dimple, cleft palate, and umbilical hernia, just to name a few. It is important to recognize that it is not enough to take a high-quality prenatal vitamin with methyl folate because so many foods we eat have been synthetically fortified with folic acid. Taking precautions to make sure that your diet, health, and genetics are cleaned up before you conceive a baby can help to drastically decrease chances of midline defects such as tongue- and lip-tie in your baby, thus enabling an easier time breastfeeding, among many other things.

Traits are strongly influenced by the environment and not just based on the genes with which you are born. For instance, height can be stunted by poor nutrition and chronic use of certain medications, and learning ability can be limited by poverty. Hundreds, if not thousands of our 20,000 genes contribute to these qualities. However, science (specifically, the study of epigenetics) is now finding that it is our environment that influences how genes express themselves.

WHAT ARE MTHFR AND GENE SNPS?

You can tell by the header that this is a slightly more complicated topic than what I've been focusing on; however, it is important, especially from a genetic perspective.

Methylenetetrahydrofolate reductase (MTHFR) is an enzyme that activates and regulates folate metabolism in the body. Specifically, MTHFR converts 5, 10- methylenetetrahydrofolate into 5-methyltetrahydrofolate (5-MTHF), the active form of folate. 5-MTHF then plays a key role in the single carbon transfer (i.e., methylation) reactions involved in the synthesis of nucleotides for DNA and RNA production; manufacture of S-adenosylmethionine (SAMe); methylation of DNA, proteins, neurotransmitters (NTs), and phospholipids; and remethylation of homocysteine to methionine.

The most well-studied, naturally occurring variants in the MTHFR gene are called C677T and A1298C. When the MTHFR gene has either of these two variants, the resulting MTHFR enzyme is slightly less active, and this can lead to decreased levels of folate and increased levels of homocysteine in the blood. It is likely that there are numerous other variations that are much rarer.

When the MTHFR genes of 564 individuals of diverse ethnicities were fully sequenced, in addition to the three common alleles mentioned above, 11 other non-synonymous changes were found, each with a frequency of 1 percent. Four of these 11 rarer alleles affected enzyme function based on tests in yeast, most of which could be fixed with higher folate supplementation (in yeast; this is not yet tested in humans). Since all five impaired alleles map to the N-terminal catalytic domain of the enzyme, it seems likely that additional single nucleotide polymorphisms (SNPs) causing non-synonymous changes in this region could have similar effects.

The Human Genome Project gave birth to the study of nutrigenomics—how nutritional status affects genetic expression and how genes affect nutrient needs. Current research in nutrigenomics indicates that some individuals, due to their unique genetic patterns and expressions, do not produce adequate or effective MTHFR. The genetic variations in DNA sequencing are known as single nucleotide polymorphisms (SNPs). When SNPs occur in genes, they produce variants or alleles of that gene. Single nucleotide polymorphisms in the gene that codes for MTHFR result in the production of an enzyme with decreased activity, an anomaly that can impact a myriad of biochemical processes. Ultimately MTHFR SNPs can cause hyperhomocysteinemia (especially if folate levels are low); affect the nervous system and behavioral and vascular health; contribute to birth defects, midline defects (tongue- and lip-tie), miscarriage and preeclampsia; modulate cancer risk; and increase chronic disease risk.

HOW DOES ENVIRONMENT AFFECT THE HEALTH OF CHILDREN?

The environment affects our health in a variety of ways. The interaction between human health and the environment has been extensively studied, and environmental risks have been proven to significantly impact human health, either directly by exposing people to harmful and toxic substances, or indirectly, by disrupting life-sustaining ecosystems. Although the exact contribution of environmental factors to the development of death and disease cannot be precisely determined, the World Health Organization (WHO) has estimated that 13 million deaths annually are attributable to preventable environmental causes. The report also estimates that 24 percent of the global disease burden (healthy life years lost) and 23 percent of all deaths (premature mortality) are attributable to environmental factors, with the environmental burden of diseases being fifteen times higher in developing countries than in developed countries, due to differences in exposure to environmental risks and access to health care.

Increasing economic development and population growth result in continuing environmental degradation. Intensification of agriculture and industrialization and increasing energy use are the most severe driving forces of environmental health problems. For countries in the early stages of development, the major environmental hazards to health are associated with widespread poverty and severe lack of public infrastructures, such as access to drinking water, sanitation, and health care, as well as emerging problems of industrial pollution.

Environmental health hazards are not limited to the developing world, although to a lesser extent, environmental risks are also present in wealthier countries and are primarily attributed to urban air and water pollution. Occurrences of asthma are rising dramatically throughout developed countries, and environmental factors appear to be at least partly to blame. The Millennium Ecosystem Assessment synthesis report warns that the erosion of ecosystems could lead to an increase in existing diseases such as malaria and cholera, as well as a rising risk of new diseases emerging.

Children are especially vulnerable to environmental threats due to their developing organs and immune systems, and their smaller bodies and airways. Harmful exposures can start as early as in utero. Furthermore, breastfeeding can be an important source of exposure to certain chemicals in infants; this should, however, not discourage breastfeeding, which carries numerous positive health and developmental benefits. Proportionate to their size, children ingest more food, drink more water, and breathe more air than adults. Additionally, certain modes of behavior, such as putting hands and objects into the mouth and playing outdoors can increase children's exposure to environmental contaminants. In short, we live in a world that is extremely toxic to our health, whether we are unborn children or more than 100 years old, and our bodies are constantly being burdened and attempting to mitigate the effects on our health.

HOW CAN MAKING BETTER CHOICES WITH HEALTH AND ENVIRONMENT RESULT IN HEALTHIER CHILDREN?

Your child's health is determined by the interaction of a multitude of influences, reflecting complex processes. Nutrition is fundamental to developing a sense of well-being and to meeting the growth, development, and activity needs of healthy, confident children and young people. Readiness to learn is enhanced when the learners are well nourished with clean, healthy foods and clean water; have a healthy, loving family unit; have proper hygiene and sleep; supplement as needed for adequate nutrition; have limited screen time; and get plenty of time outside for play.

Food and nutrition play an essential role in children's and young people's achievement at all stages of education. There is evidence that young people's food choices can affect their behavior as well as their health. Part of the role of early childhood education services and schools is to provide an environment where students learn, and this includes learning to make healthy food choices. Early childhood education and school settings provide numerous, diverse opportunities for children and young people to make decisions about food, which is why it is vital that these environments are structured to promote and support healthy eating.

WHAT DOES IT ALL MEAN?

My husband and I both have different MTHFR genetic mutations that we've passed down to our children. I was aware of this before they were born, which enabled me to make choices that would ultimately prevent certain traits associated with MTHFR. These genes can be turned on or off in unborn babies! This knowledge is powerful in preventing disease and ill health within our families. It doesn't necessarily mean you have to run out and test everyone in your family, but it does mean that cleaning up your genes with diet and lifestyle choices will prevent the expression of certain diseases.

Genetics and epigenetics explain different phenotypic changes in traits of different organisms with the evolution of modern science. Genetics is a pathway of science concentrated on the study of genes, heredity, and genetic variations of living organisms. Gregor Mendel explained that different traits of an organism are passed from one generation to the next by genes. Over time, different experiments revealed that DNA is the molecule responsible for inheritance, where the genetic information is passed to the next generation. Genetics initiated the study of different subcategories, such as epigenetics. Epigenetics refers to the development of different heritable traits due to the influence of external factors like diet, lifestyle, behavioral patterns, and environmental conditions.

What is the major take-home point? As much as humanly possible, change your lifestyle, clean up your diet and environments, fix your gut and microbiome, and deal with emotional stressors. If you do this, you will have dramatic health changes you never thought possible. Resist the need to feel you are a victim to your "genetics." Science is now understanding that our genes change the way they "express" themselves based on our environment.

THE GERM THEORY

We live in a germy world. Germs are everywhere. Everyday expressions are that we "catch a cold" or "we caught the flubug." But what more should be taken into consideration?

The germ theory of disease is based on the concept that many diseases are caused by infections with microorganisms, typically only visualized under high magnification. Such microorganisms can consist of bacterial, viral, fungal, or protist species. Although the growth and productive replication of microorganisms are the cause of disease, environmental and genetic factors may predispose a host or influence the severity of the infection. For example, in an immune-compromised host (e.g., due to AIDS or old age), an infection may result in more severe outcomes than in individuals who are fully immunocompetent.

Proving the germ theory of disease was the crowning achievement of the French scientist Louis Pasteur. Born in Dole, Eastern France, Pasteur was a conscientious, hard-working student, though not considered exceptional. One of his professors called him "mediocre." He received a doctorate in 1847, and after obtaining posts at Strasbourg, Lille, and Paris, he spent much time researching aspects of chemistry.

His most important discoveries were in the field of germ study. When Pasteur set out to understand the fermentation process, he discovered that alcohol in wine was produced by yeast which lived on the skins of grapes. During fermentation, the yeast appeared healthy and budding under a microscope, but lactic acid was formed and the wine turned to vinegar as other microbes were seen among the yeast cells. Further analysis of the wine showed a number of complex organic molecules, some of which were able to rotate light, a property of compounds produced by living organisms. Through several experiments, Pasteur showed that fermentation required contact with dust in the air.

Pasteur then turned his attention to the health of silkworms, which produced silk for the cloth industry. He discovered that healthy silkworms became ill when they nested in the bedding of those suffering from disease. In this study, Pasteur found that environment directly affected contagion and that the spread of disease could be controlled by sterilization. His studies on yeast had shown that microbes could be airborne, and he realized that these two studies could be directly applied to the transmission of disease in humans.

The final proof of germ theory came when Pasteur was able to grow the anthrax bacillus in culture. Although anthrax had been isolated by Robert Koch, opponents believed that the spores he found could have been contaminants in his culture medium. Pasteur placed a drop of blood from a sheep dying of anthrax into a sterile culture and allowed the bacilli to grow. He repeated this process until none of the original cultures remained in the final dish. The final culture produced anthrax when injected into sheep, showing that the bacillus was responsible for the disease.

One of his most radical achievements was developing practical ways of killing bacteria in liquids, such as milk. His process of pasteurization successfully killed bacteria in milk without destroying milk protein. This was a radical discovery and made drinking milk safe. The process of pasteurization was named after him, and it saved many lives.

Louis Pasteur was a great believer in hard work. Never content to rest on his laurels, he continued to work very hard in his laboratory to develop more cures. In 1860 the French Academy announced a prize of 2,500 francs to anyone who provided convincing experimental proof for or against spontaneous generation of life.

Pasteur was awarded the prize in 1862. He showed that no microbes ever grew in nutrient solutions that had been sterilized by heating, provided the air above the solutions was also sterilized. If unsterilized air was allowed into the space above the solutions, microbes began growing in the solutions.

The Pasteur Institute opened in 1888. During Louis Pasteur's lifetime, it was not easy for him to convince others of his ideas, which were controversial in their time but considered absolutely correct today. Pasteur fought to convince surgeons that germs existed and carried diseases, and that dirty instruments and hands spread germs and therefore disease.

Pasteur's pasteurization process killed germs and prevented the spread of disease. He found a cure for rabies and for anthrax. His principles were used by scientists in developing vaccines for disease, such as typhus, diphtheria, cholera, yellow fever, and different strains of plague.

Louis Pasteur had great faith in the good nature of humans. He worked tirelessly to deliver real benefits for the treatment of infectious diseases. More than any other person, Louis Pasteur helped to increase the average life expectancy in the late nineteenth and early twentieth centuries.

WHY IS THE GERM THEORY CONTROVERSIAL?

According to Louis Pasteur's widely accepted germ theory, many illnesses and diseases are carried by microorganisms from which we must protect ourselves. Conversely, the human gastrointestinal tract, for example, harbors trillions of microbes and couldn't function without them. Well then, which is it? Are bacteria friend or enemy?

Let us revisit the germ theory. If we are at the mercy of these little bad guys called bacteria and viruses in our environment, then why aren't we all affected? Have you ever wondered why a group of people exposed to an equal measure of the same germs respond differently? Take the recent appearance of swine flu, for instance. Why did some die, some get sick and then better, and others were unaffected altogether? If we were truly at the mercy of this virus, wouldn't we all be dead? As extreme as this may sound, we must ask why some people are affected and others untouched. Is it bad luck? Is it sheer chance? Or are there other factors at play here?

Germs are scientifically classified as opportunistic species. This means that they can only "attack" if and only if they are given the opportunity, which means in a weak host or a person with a weakened immune system. If your immune system is weak, you have now become a target; you are now an opportunity. This can easily be seen in the increased susceptibility of the elderly, the very young, or in extreme cases, people with AIDS. For example, an AIDS patient can die from the common cold due to the decreased function of the immune system. So are germs really the culprit? Are we victims of germs? Or are we victims of a weakened immune system? This is why this theory is, if nothing else, incomplete.

WHAT IS THE HOST THEORY?

In nineteenth-century France, while Pasteur was advocating the notion of germs as the cause of disease, another French scientist named Antoine Béchamp advocated a conflicting theory known as the "cellular theory" of disease – now referred to as the "Host Theory."

In the host theory, people don't "catch" germs that give them diseases. Instead, disease-causing germs are actually opportunistic, thriving in people whose bodies have a weakness or who are imbalanced internally. They are a by-product of the disease, not a cause of the disease. We have viruses, and bacteria in and on us all the time, every second! A healthy balance of beneficial bacteria and a healthy body environment keep the unhealthy stuff out and in balance. For example, if we kill off everything by using antibacterial soaps all the time or by taking antibiotics for every little cold, then we aren't just destroying the bad bacteria, we are radically wiping out all the beneficial bacteria as well, leaving us even more susceptible to new diseases in the long run.

Pierre Jacques Antoine Béchamp (October 16, 1816 to April 15, 1908) was a French scientist now best known for breakthroughs in applied organic chemistry and for a bitter rivalry with Louis Pasteur. Béchamp had an incredible list of scientist appointments at French universities, receiving a doctor of science degree in 1853 and doctor of medicine in 1856; professor of medical chemistry and pharmacy at Montpelier, and professor of physics and toxicology at Strasbourg. He also ran a pharmacy in the city.

During his lifetime, Béchamp was overshadowed by the iconic chemist Louis Pasteur (1822–1895), the most celebrated scientist of the nineteenth century. He is considered the father of medical microbiology, and some call him the father of modern medicine, a title quite remarkable, especially because Pasteur was not a physician. Both men were highly regarded members of the French Academy of Science, and each submitted their scientific findings to the academy for review and publication.

Because Béchamp frequently criticized Pasteur's work, an intense rivalry and feud between the two intensified in the academy. No matter how carefully Béchamp argued against some of Pasteur's scientific methods and conclusions, the academy always gave the nod to Pasteur.

Béchamp's cellular theory is almost completely opposite that of Pasteur's. Béchamp noted that these germs that so terrified Pasteur were opportunistic in nature. They were everywhere and even existed inside us in a symbiotic relationship. Béchamp noticed in his research that it was only when the tissue of the host became damaged or compromised that these germs began to manifest as a prevailing symptom (not cause) of disease.

To prevent illness, Béchamp advocated not the killing of germs but the cultivation of health through diet, hygiene, and healthy lifestyle practices such as getting fresh air and exercise. The idea is that if the person has a strong immune system and good tissue quality (or "terrain," as Béchamp called it), the germs will not manifest in the person, and they will have good health. It is only when their health starts to decline (due to personal neglect and poor lifestyle choices) that they fall victim to infectious diseases.

To treat illness, Béchamp's cellular theory also applied. Béchamp was less concerned with killing the infection than he was with restoring the health of the patient's body through healthy lifestyle choices. Béchamp saw the infection as a footnote to the state of illness and not the primary cause. As the person's health was restored through diet, hygiene, and detoxification, the infection went away on its own—without needing measures to kill it.

Pasteur and Béchamp had a long, often bitter rivalry regarding who was right about the true cause of illness. Ultimately Pasteur's ideas were accepted by society, and Béchamp was pretty much forgotten. The practice of Western medicine is based on Pasteur's germ theory, which gives rise to the use of vaccinations, antibiotics, and other antimicrobials.

The irony is that toward the end of his life, Pasteur renounced the germ theory and admitted that Béchamp was right all along. Moreover, in the 1920s, medical historians discovered that most of Pasteur's theories were plagiarized from Béchamp's early research work. Béchamp is a doctor of science, doctor of medicine, professor of medical chemistry and pharmacy at Montpelier, and professor of physics and toxicology at Strasbourg. In 1854 Béchamp was appointed professor of chemistry at the University of Strasbourg, a post previously held by Louis Pasteur.

Béchamp developed the Béchamp reduction, an inexpensive method to produce aniline dye, permitting Perkin (who created the first synthetic dye in 1856) to launch the synthetic-dye industry. Béchamp also synthesized the first organic arsenical drug, arsanilic acid, from which Ehrlich later synthesized the first chemotherapeutic drug. Béchamp's rivalry with Pasteur was initially for priority in attributing fermentation to microorganisms, later for attributing the silkworm disease pebrine to microorganisms, and eventually over the validity of germ theory. Béchamp also disputed cell theory.

Claiming discovery that the "molecular granulations" in biological fluids were actually the elementary units of life, Béchamp named them microzymas, or "tiny enzymes, "and credited them with producing both enzymes and cells while "evolving" amid favorable conditions into multicellular organisms. Denying that bacteria could invade a healthy animal and cause disease, Béchamp claimed instead that unfavorable host and environmental conditions destabilize the host's native microzymas, whereupon they decompose host tissue by producing pathogenic bacteria. While cell theory and germ theory gained widespread acceptance, granular theories became obscure. Béchamp's version, microzymian theory, has been retained by small groups, especially in alternative medicine.

Unlike Pasteur, who spawned a mentality of killing germs to prevent disease, Béchamp understood the importance of the internal environment that is created with proper food choices, good hygiene, and other healthy lifestyle habits. He was an early proponent of the concept that making different choices with our health will either support or resist disease.

Béchamp theorized that germs were actually the chemical by-products and the degenerative aspects of the unbalanced state of a body. For the disease to take hold, cellular miscommunication, dysfunction, and dead tissue had to already be occurring in the body. That's when the germ or bacteria shows up and sets up shop because the body (or an area of the body) is in a state that lets them thrive and gives them a home. This cellular dysfunction or dead tissue is caused by malnutrition or exposure to toxins.

As you can see, host theory and germ theory are two radically different views of how people acquire disease.

GERMS AND THE HUMAN GENOME

The human genome is made up of about 23,000 genes. That's an impressive figure, until you consider that the number of nonhuman genes that each of us carries around from the bacteria, viruses, and other pathogens living in and on us totals eight million. Most of the cells in the human body aren't human. Indeed, bacterial cells outnumber human cells at a 10 to 1 ratio, which is why the exploration of the human microbiomes (the collective population of all the nonhuman cells and genes that inhabit us) is currently one of the fastest rising fields of medical research.

What scientists are discovering is that these microbes are not just freeloaders or invaders. Rather, they're crucial facilitators of many of our basic bodily functions—from digesting food and producing vitamins to fending off harmful infections and recovering from illnesses. They not only keep people healthy, but they may also explain differences in individual health—why people respond differently to the same drug or why some people develop chronic diseases and others do not.

Depending on what may be living in it or mixed into it, food, water, or air can become dangerous to humans and other animals. When this happens, it is said to be contaminated or polluted. Food and water can be contaminated by disease-causing germs.

Germs can get into the body through the mouth, nose, breaks in the skin, eyes, and genitals. Once disease-causing germs are inside the body, they can stop it from working properly. They may breed very quickly, and in a very short amount of time, a small number of germs can become millions. However, there are many germs inside the human body that may not cause disease. Some even help parts of the body work properly. For example, the gut cannot digest food properly without the help of certain "good" bacteria.

In closing, my own personal experience with the germ theory is that we need to be clean but not germaphobic. At many points in my life I have been fearful of "germs" in my environment. I always have to remind myself that the terrain or environment in which we live is so important, but we need to make lifestyle choices that are focused on clean eating, pure water, exercise, stress reduction, and a hopeful attitude to create a healthier immune system, and therefore a healthier host.

Living in this mindful way creates an environment in which diseases cannot thrive and can yield a healthy, long life full of vitality.

OUR TOXIC HOMES

We are exposed to an overwhelming number of chemicals/toxins every day that enter our body via ingestion, inhalation, or absorption through the skin. We are adding to this toxic burden through the regular use of cleaning products and detergents. The chemicals from these products enter the bloodstream and require detoxification by the liver for removal, placing extra stress on the liver and supporting organs to filter out the toxins. The majority of these toxins are fat-soluble and can be stored in fat or muscle tissue for years. Although occasional exposure to these chemicals may not have a profound effect, long-term, repetitive exposure increases the risk of toxicity and adverse health outcomes.

The average household will have approximately 250 to 300 chemicals in the form of cleaning products, garden products, handyman products, or detergents. Some of these chemicals have such severe acute toxicity that they necessitate treatment in the emergency department for chemical burns or accidental ingestion. In many parts of the world, including

Australia, there are poor government regulations to control which chemicals (or how many) are put into these products.

Keep in mind that most household cleaning products and pesticides are reasonably safe when used as directed and that a product's level of toxicity is dependent on the dose of the product used (never use more than the amount listed on the label) and the length of exposure to the product.

When consumers buy commercial cleaning products, we expect them to do one thing: clean! We use a wide array of scents, soaps, detergents, bleaching agents, softeners, scourers, polishes, and specialized cleaners for bathrooms, glass, drains, and ovens to keep our homes sparkling and sweet-smelling. But while the chemicals in cleaners disinfect our dishes, bathtubs, and countertops and make them gleam, many contribute to indoor air pollution, are poisonous if ingested, and can be harmful if inhaled or touched. In fact, some cleaners are among the most toxic products found in the home. In 2000, cleaning products were responsible for nearly 10 percent (accounting for 206,636 calls) of all toxic exposures reported to U.S. Poison Control Centers. Of those calls, more than half (120,434 exposures) involved children under six who had swallowed or spilled cleaners stored or left open inside the home.

The type of health hazards that cleaning ingredients pose varies. Some cause acute (immediate) reactions such as skin or respiratory irritation, watery eyes, or chemical burns, while others are associated with chronic (long-term) effects such as cancer.

The most acutely dangerous cleaning products are corrosive drain cleaners, oven cleaners, and acidic toilet-bowl cleaners, according to Philip Dickey of the Washington Toxics Coalition. Corrosive chemicals can cause severe burns to the eyes and skin, and if ingested, to the throat and esophagus as well. Ingredients with high acute toxicity include chlorine bleach and ammonia, which produce fumes that are highly irritating to the eyes, nose, throat, and lungs and should not be used by people with asthma or suffering from lung or heart problems. These two chemicals pose an added threat in that they can react with each other or other chemicals to form lung-damaging gases.

With that said, you can be confident that the cleaning products you buy are thoroughly assessed to ensure they are safe to use. By law, manufacturers must make sure the products they sell are safe, provided they are used correctly and according to the instructions. If a product is found to be unsafe, manufacturers must take it off the market.

When thinking about safety, it is important to understand the difference between hazard and risk. A hazard is something that can cause harm; a risk is the chance that it will cause harm.

To make sure products are safe to use, cleaning-product manufacturers examine the toxicity of every ingredient. They calculate what dose someone might receive when using the product, through each route of exposure: skin contact, breathing in vapor, even ingestion of residues. They make sure there are wide margins of safety between the possible dose and one that could cause harm.

WHAT DOES THE RESEARCH SHOW?

The soap and cleaning-compound manufacturing industry in the United States, which produces such household products as laundry detergents, lime/rust removers, and various other all-purpose cleaners, was forecast to generate about $61.06 billion by 2016. A household cleaner has to be effective, gentle on users, and have a nice scent. Beneath your sink you likely have a wide variety of cleaning products, some that you use every day and others you rarely use. Manufacturers want to be sure that their product is not only safe, but that it is also the one your reach for most often. Every household cleaner requires optimal combinations of ingredients (e.g., surfactants, stain removers, brighteners, abrasives, and sanitizers) to ensure peak performance, BUT it also needs to be gentle on users' hands and appeal to their senses.

Household cleaners, paints, and perfumes have become substantial sources of urban air pollution. Researchers in the U.S. looked at levels of synthetic Volatile Organic Compounds (VOCs) in the roadside air in Los Angeles and found that as much came from industrial and household products refined from petroleum as from vehicle exhaust pipes.

The compounds are an essential contributor to air pollution because when they drift into the atmosphere, they react with other chemicals to produce harmful ozone or fine particulate matter known as PM2.5. Ground-level ozone can trigger breathing problems by making the airways constrict, while fine airborne particles drive heart and lung disease.

Also, women who worked in dry cleaners suffered lung damage similar to what someone would experience by smoking 20 cigarettes a day. Women who cleaned on a regular basis as part of their job were affected the most, followed by women who clean at home; lastly, women who were affected the least were those who didn't clean much at all.

Household cleaners, including some labeled as "natural," contain chemicals that are hazardous to human health, according to a new report from the Environmental Working Group (EWG), a research and advocacy group in areas of agriculture subsidies, chemicals, and pollutants. Research conducted by the EWG showed that household cleaning products available in the U.S. might contain compounds banned in other countries that are known to cause blindness, cancer, asthma, and other severe conditions. These cleaners may present severe risks to children who may ingest them, spill them, or breathe their fumes, according to the EWG.

WHICH CLEANING PRODUCTS ARE DANGEROUS TO OUR HEALTH?

Scientists now realize the chemicals found in a wide array of household goods are more toxic than previously thought. Since health and wellness are not simply about diet and exercise, but also about limiting exposure to toxicity, it is important to become aware of these items and to take action to remove them wherever possible.

Antifreeze. Ethylene glycol, the main hazardous ingredient in antifreeze, is extremely poisonous. Iinhalation of the fumes can cause dizziness, swallowing antifreeze will cause severe damage to the heart, kidneys, and brain; indeed, it can be fatal.

Laundry detergents: These products contain enzymes (as noted by the names "cationic," "anionic," or "non-ionic" on the label) to loosen stains and ground-in dirt. Cationic detergents are the most toxic when taken internally. Ingestion can result in nausea, vomiting, shock, convulsions, and coma. Non-ionic detergents are less toxic but can irritate the skin and eyes or make you more sensitive to other chemicals. Asthma can develop if a person is exposed to large quantities of detergent. Detergents are also responsible for many household poisonings due to accidental swallowing.

Insecticides: Insecticides contain some of the same pesticides found in pet flea and tick treatments. In addition to permethrin, other pesticide chemicals commonly found in insecticides are diazinon, propoxur, and chlorpyrifos, which can cause headache, dizziness, twitching, and nausea.

Antibacterial cleaners: Antibacterial cleaners usually contain water, a fragrance, a surfactant (to break up dirt), and a pesticide. The pesticides commonly used in antibacterial cleaners are quaternary ammonium or phenolic chemicals. Antibacterial cleaners can irritate your eyes and burn your skin and throat.

Antiperspirants: Most people wear antiperspirant to prevent body odor, but one of the "sweat-blocking" ingredients found in many antiperspirants is aluminum. In recent years, questions have been raised about whether the aluminum in antiperspirants can contribute to the development of breast cancer and Alzheimer's disease. While the studies are inconclusive, the U.S. Food and Drug Administration requires a warning label on all antiperspirants.

Cosmetics: The average person applies between six and 12 cosmetic items per day, and most of these will include toxic chemicals that are potentially harmful. It is always a good idea to look for cosmetics that are free of synthetic fragrances and that are mineral-based or made from natural oils. Buying organic products can help greatly reduce your exposure to toxins.

Plastic drinking bottles: We are all aware by now that plastic bottles are not great for the environment, but they can also leak toxic chemicals into your drink. Most bottles are now BPA-free, which is a step in the right direction. However, that is not the only harmful chemical in plastics, so it's always safer to use a glass or steel container when you can.

Plastic food containers: Many plastic containers are made from chemicals such as phthalates, which can interfere with the body's endocrine system and produce adverse developmental, reproductive, and neurological effects in humans; in addition, since the plastic breaks down over time, it can cause the release of these dangerous chemicals into your food. Switch to glass containers wherever possible. In my opinion, there is no such thing as "safe plastic."

Air fresheners/scented candles: Like cleaning products, air fresheners help keep our homes nice, but a study by the University of California at Berkeley found that when used excessively or in an unventilated area, they release toxic levels of pollutants. Having air fresheners around your home should not make you sick, but you must ensure the area is ventilated to stop the toxic chemicals (e.g., ethylene-based glycol ethers and paradichlorobenzene) from circulating through the air and adversely impacting your health.

Perfumes: A study by the Environmental Protection Agency found that potentially hazardous chemicals can commonly be found in fragrances. Toxic chemicals like benzaldehyde, camphor, ethyl acetate, benzyl acetate, linalool, acetone, and methylene chloride can, when inhaled, cause dizziness; nausea; drowsiness; irritation to the throat, eyes, skin, and lungs; kidney damage; and headaches.

Canned food: BisphenolA (BPA), found in most canned food containers, is a hormone-disrupting chemical linked to infertility, heart disease, and diabetes. Although some manufacturers are phasing the chemical out of their cans, it's not clear that the replacements are safe either. If possible, opt for fresh or frozen foods.

TOXIC, HAZARDOUS OR BOTH

Chemicals are toxic if they can harm us when they enter or contact the body. Since chemicals can be toxic, it is essential to understand how they can affect our health. To determine the risk of harmful health effects from a substance, you must first know how toxic the substance is; how much and by what means a person is exposed; and how sensitive that person is to the substance.

Exposure to a toxic substance such as gasoline can affect your health. For example, drinking gasoline can cause burns, vomiting, diarrhea, and in very large amounts, drowsiness or death. Some chemicals are hazardous because of their physical properties: they can explode, burn, or react easily with other chemicals. Since gasoline can burn and its vapors can explode, gasoline is also hazardous. A chemical can be toxic, hazardous, or both.

Thankfully, our bodies are designed to detoxify. However, when external sources of toxicity are added to the mix, those normal detoxification processes become overwhelmed and therefore do not work as well. External toxins add to the "total body load" or "total body burden." The liver is the body's main detoxification organ. A fully functional liver supports immune system function. The immune system is part of your body's detoxification arsenal and part of the machinery that protects you from toxins. It is constantly struggling to keep up. Toxins cause free radicals that bind to cytokines (information pathways), causing a breakdown in vital immune information flow.

There comes a time when a person's immune system just cannot handle any more insults and becomes completely overwhelmed. Best described by the "straw that broke the camel's back," this concept most often refers to the point in time when a person shifts into autoimmunity.

Detoxification is something we need to consider. Whether detoxing your body with juice fasts, eliminating BPAs, or choosing only organic products—from beauty supplies to food and clothing—more people than ever are concerned about what is going into our homes and our bodies. Despite the renewed attention, plenty of toxins remain in products we use every day, especially common household cleaning products, which can have dire health effects.

WHAT DO TOXIC CLEANING PRODUCTS DO TO OUR ENDOCRINE SYSTEM?

Endocrine disruptors are chemicals that may interfere with the production or activity of hormones in the human endocrine system. These chemicals may occur naturally or be manufactured. The term "endocrine disruptors" describes a diverse group of chemicals that are suspected of affecting or known to affect human hormones. Effects on human hormones can range from minor to serious, depending on the specific endocrine receptor and the amount of exposure. Because these chemicals are found in products you use every day and you are exposed to many endocrine disruptors at the same time, it is difficult to determine the public health effects of these chemicals.

The human endocrine system is responsible for controlling and coordinating many bodily functions, including the production of hormones. The human endocrine system includes the pancreas, pituitary, thyroid, adrenal, and male and female reproductive glands.

Endocrine disruptors interfere with the production, release, transport, metabolism, or elimination of the body's natural hormones. They can mimic naturally occurring hormones, potentially causing overproduction or underproduction of hormones. They may also interfere with or block the way natural hormones and their receptors are made or controlled.

Today, the amount of highly toxic chemicals with which our society is saturated is almost inconceivable. Exposure to synthetic chemicals is a given in today's world. They are in the air we breathe, the food we eat, the products we apply to our skin, and the mattresses on which we sleep. Mounting research indicates that they are in our blood and urine as well.

TOXIC CLEANING PRODUCTS AND LUNG ISSUES

Regular use of cleaning sprays has an impact on lung health comparable with smoking a pack of cigarettes every day, according to a new study. The research followed more than 6,000 people over a 20-year period and found that women in particular suffered significant health problems after long-term use of these products.

Lung-function decline in women working as cleaners or regularly using cleaning products at home was comparable to smoking 20 cigarettes a day over 10 to 20 years. The scientists who carried out the study advised that such products should be avoided and can generally be replaced with simple microfiber cloths and water.

According to the American Lung Association (ALA), some chemicals in cleaning products, such as ammonia and bleach, are already known to contribute to respiratory problems and accidentally mixing a product containing ammonia with one that contains bleach can produce a dangerous gas that can be deadly if inhaled. For this reason, the ALA, as well as other health organizations, recommends minimal exposure to these products. However, this new study is the first to show a link between cleaning products and chronic obstructive pulmonary disease (COPD) specifically among health-care workers.

Chronic obstructive pulmonary disease (COPD) is a medical term covering progressive lung conditions such as emphysema, chronic bronchitis, nonreversible asthma, and some forms of bronchiectasis. Each of these diseases is characterized by an increasing difficulty with breathing or "catching your breath." Breathlessness and coughing are not normal symptoms of aging, but are rather symptoms of a progressive disease that may ultimately claim your life.

Individuals who suffer from diseases that fall under the umbrella term of COPD may experience frequent wheezing, coughing, and chest tightness, as well as increasing breathlessness. Diseases that fall under the umbrella term of COPD touch the lives of nearly 30 million people in the U.S., many of whom are unaware they are affected. According to the COPD Foundation, these conditions may be triggered by smoking, secondhand smoke, fumes, and chemicals such as found in cleaning products.

WHY HAVE I NOT BEEN INFORMED ABOUT THESE TOXIC CLEANING PRODUCTS?

Have you ever considered how odd it is that there are warning labels on cleaning products? I mean, think about that: they're supposed to be ridding your home of bad stuff, not adding to it, much less they are not supposed to be potentially making you sick! A good stand-up comedian could build an entire act from this one bizarre fact.

And here's something even less amusing: The labels on cleaning products do not tell you about most of the toxic ingredients they contain. If these products are as safe as they claim to be, why don't the companies tell us what's in them? Call me suspicious, but I honestly do not think it is because the recipe is top secret. If it were, there would not be so many competing products with identical ingredients.

Do not look to the government for help on this one. The government only requires companies to list "chemicals of known concern" on their labels. The key word here is "known." The fact is that the government has no idea whether most of the chemicals used in everyday cleaning products are safe because it does not test them, and it does not require manufacturers to test them either.

Actually, under the terms of the Toxic Substances Control Act of 1976, the U.S. Environmental Protection Agency (EPA), which administers the act, cannot require chemical companies to prove the safety of their products unless the agency itself can show the product poses a health risk—which the EPA does not have the resources to do since, according to one estimate, it receives some 2,000 new applications for approval every year. How tough is their review? You decide: in 2003, according to the Environmental Working Group, an agency watchdog, the EPA approved most applications in three weeks, even though more than half had provided no information on toxicity at all.

This means that we must use the same vigilance in selecting the products we use to clean and store in our homes as we do in maintaining our other health requirements, including nutrition, exercise, sleep, attitude, and environment.

For a list of toxic cleaning products, please refer to Appendix D.

EPILOGUE

The road to healing can be hard and include a lot of suffering, but we can also choose to see it in a different light. Our healing can be our greatest teacher and bring about greater awareness on a physical, mental, and emotional level. By asking different questions, listening to your body and following natures simple laws, healing from within is attainable for everyone. Health is our birthright. My hope is that the topics discussed in this book make your health journey easier and more straightforward.

My intention in writing this book was to elevate your conscious awareness that your body is truly amazing and wants to Heal from Within. If you have found the information in this book interesting and helpful, please let others know so that they, too, can be helped on this journey. Leaving a positive review also helps others take a step toward a healthier future.

I want you to decide what it means to become truly healthy. One thing for certain is that unless we are sick or in pain, we often do not think about or ask about our health. In our culture, we believe that if we feel good and look good (or at least if we do not feel pain), we must be healthy. I hope that now, after reading this book, you fully understand the definition of health, which is "wholeness or optimal function."

My vision is that our country will raise its standards on health, but until that happens, you can heighten your awareness and take your health and the health of your children into your own hands. When the day is done, it's your fate after all.

Here's to your happy, healthy future!

THANK YOU FOR READING

ADDITIONAL INFORMATION, REFERRALS AND RESOURCES

APPENDIX A: LOCAL RESOURCES

The following include the individual name, company name, address and/or contact number of all the local companies and health care providers that I know personally, have worked with, or for whom my patients have offered rave reviews. I love supporting local businesses, so if you are reading this book and you are in the St. Louis area, know that you have some amazing resources to tap into. These are also on my website where they will be updated periodically: www.keoughchiropratic.com.

Family Medicine

Michael Schoenwalder, DO
1585 Woodlake Dr. #104
Chesterfield, MO 63017
(314) 721-2140

Webster Family Physicians
Christian Wessling, MD
Family Practice Physician
7979 Big Bend Blvd.
St. Louis, MO 63119
(314) 961-6631

Acupuncture

Caitlin Cross, DC
Keough Chiropractic
2440 Executive Drive
St. Charles, MO 63303

Dr. Liu
Authentic Chinese Herbs & Acupuncture Co.
8144-46 Olive Blvd.
University City, MO 63130
(314) 567-6443

Bryan Harasha
Center for Mind Body Spirit
7649 Delmar Blvd.
St. Louis, MO 63130

OB-GYN

Obstetrical Associates, Inc.
Laura I. Moore, MD
224 S. Woods Mill Rd.
Chesterfield, MO 63017
(314) 576-9797

Laura Laue, DO
Obstetrician-Gynecologist
12277 De Paul Dr. #305
Bridgeton, MO 63044
(314) 344-7585

Loria A. Lindsey, MD
Obstetrician-Gynecologist
20 Progress Point Pkwy.
O'Fallon, MO 63368
(636) 926-0404

Emanuel J. Vlastos, MD (V-BAC)
Family Practice Physician
1031 Bellevue Ave. #400
St. Louis, MO 63117
(314) 977-7455

Sandra Minchow Proffitt, MD
Family Practice Physician
Mercy Family Medicine
12680 Olive Blvd. # 300
St. Louis, MO 63141
(314) 251-8888

Jeffrey Mormol, MD
555 North New Ballas, Ste. 240
Creve Coeur, MO 63141

Midwives

Birth and Wellness Center
769 W. Terra Ln.
O'Fallon, MO 63366
(636) 294-6441

Mercy Birth Center – St. Louis

615 South New Ballas Rd.,
Ste. 1400

St. Louis, MO 63141

(314) 251-7955

Julie Guttman (home birth midwife)

(314) 608-9854

Allison Doughtery
(home birth midwife)

(314) 805-7202

Jen Jester

(314) 374-8901

www.birthwisely.net

birthwisely@gmail.com

Doulas

Jamie Bodily

(636) 699-2839

Andrea Meintz

(314) 578-3317

Barb Hueffmeier

(636) 795-8481

Samanda Rossi

(314) 225-7891

Emma Ginder

(217) 691-2216

Marissa Barbeau

(314) 477-1642

Jamie Bodily

(314) 399-8457

Haley Manning

(617) 595-5123

Jenny Woodman

(314) 477-1642

Kaityn Seabacher

(636) 328-8971

Fertility Methods/ Ovulation Tracking

Creighton Model –
www.creightonmodel.com/

Billings Method –
www.billingsmethod.com/

Marquette Method –
nfp.marquette.edu/

Placenta Encapsulation

Teresa Goodlett

(314) 303-8257

Lisa Norton VanDyne

636-699-2217

Alicia Brooks

http://www.yourjoyfulbirth.com/

Lactation Consultants

Kadie Tannehill

(314) 258-6963

Johanna Iwaszkowiek

(773) 354-1853

Molly Ottolini

(636) 236-1852

Kangaroo Kids

(314) 835-9200

Female/Pregnancy Support Garments

Hanger Clinic: Orthotic & Prosthetic Solutions

150 St. Peters Center Blvd., Ste. A

St. Peters, MO 63376

(636) 922-3260

Hanger Clinic: Orthotics & Prosthetics Service

9719 Olive Blvd.

Olivette, MO 63132

(314) 567-6844

Holistic Dentists

C. Lee Row and
Gregory A. Pucel, DDS

510 Baxter Rd. #3

Chesterfield, MO 63017

(636) 391-1911

Michael G. Rehme, DDS, CCN and Associates

2821 N. Ballas Rd. #245

St. Louis, MO 63131

(314) 997-2550

Cherry Hills Dental

Rodney Lofton, DDS

16976 Manchester Rd.

Grover, MO 63040

(636) 458-9090

Pediatricians who allow delayed vaccine schedule

Little Flowers Family Medicine

207 E. Pitman St.

O'Fallon, MO 63366

(636) 875-1140

Randy Agolia, MD
20 Progress Point Parkway #220
O'Fallon, MO 63368
Mosaic Family Medicine

Sandra Minchow Proffitt, MD
(TEMPORARY LOCATION)
3844 S. Lindbergh Blvd., Suite 200
Sunset Hills, MO 63127

Dr. Anu French – Pediatrician (www.anufrench.com)
DePaul Health Center
12255 DePaul Drive
Bridgeton, MO 63044

Occupational Therapists

Play to Learn
14360 South Outer Forty Drive
Chesterfield, MO 63017
(314) 434-5410

Leaps and Bounds
324 Jungermann Rd.
St. Peters, MO 63376
(636) 928-5327

Brain Balance Center
6133 Mid Rivers Mall Dr.
St Peters, MO 63304
636-685-0333

Massage Therapy

Sadie Keough, LMT
2440 Executive Drive, Ste. 102
St. Charles, MO 63303
(636) 219-0111

Christie Blaise, LMT
2440 Executive Drive, Ste. 102
St. Charles, MO 63303
(636) 219-7930

Physical Therapists

Kevin J. Wilhite, PT
2394 State Hwy. K
O'Fallon, MO 63368
(636) 978-3711

Legacy Physical Therapy, LLC
The Shoppes At Seven Oaks
2961 Dougherty Ferry Rd., Suite 105
St. Louis, MO 63122
(636) 225-3649

Atletico Physical Therapy
(Multiple locations in St. Louis/ St. Charles MO)

Orthopedics

Orthopedic Center of St Louis
Kaylea M. Boutwell, MD
14825 N. Outer 40 Rd. #200
Chesterfield, MO 63017
(314) 336-2555

US Sports Medicine
Rick Lehman, MD
333 South Kirkwood Rd, Ste 200
St. Louis, MO 63122
(314) 909-1666

Advanced Bone and Joint
Paul M. Spezia, DO
Brandon D. Larkin, MD
Brian D. Meek, MD
W. Anthony Frisella, MD
112 Piper Hill Dr. #9
St. Peters, MO 63376
(636) 229-4222

Piper Spine Care
112 Piper Hill Dr., Ste. 6
St Peters MO 63376
(636) 229-5900

St. Charles Orthopedic Surgery
Kevin J. Quigley, MD
5301 Veterans Memorial Pkwy.
St. Peters, MO 63376
(636) 561-0871

Jones & Sciortino Orthopedics (hip surgeon)
224 S. Woods Mill Rd.
Chesterfield, MO 63017
(314) 434-3240

Paul Young, MD
St. Anthony's Hospital
10012 Kennerly Rd., Suite 400
St. Louis, MO 63128
(314) 543-5999

Kurt Eichholz, MD
4590 S. Lindbergh Blvd.
St. Louis, MO 63127
(314) 270-9494

Podiatrist

Paranjge Amod, DPM
3701 N. St. Peters Pkwy., Ste. C
St. Peters, MO
(636) 442-1541

Magdalena Lafontant , DPM
Foot Healers
St. Peters, MO
(636) 279-1900

Dermatologists

Natalie L. Semchyshyn, MD

Dermatologist

2315 Dougherty Ferry Rd. #200C

St. Louis, MO 63131

(314) 977-9666

Holistic Skin Care

Esthetician Service

Jayme Hanna

Birch Botanical Spa

2440 Executive Drive, Ste. 102

St. Charles, MO 63303

birchbotanicalspa.com

Counseling Services (smoking, fears, diet, weight loss, PTSD)

Family Life Counseling & Psychological Services, LLC

4142 Keaton Crossing Blvd., Ste. 101

O'Fallon, MO 63368

(636) 300-9333

Tracy Turner-Bumberry, LPC

Family Counselor

428 McDonough St. #201

Saint Charles, MO 63301

(636) 724-1224

Albers Mind and Body Wellness

5988 Mid Rivers Mall Dr.

St. Peters, MO 63304

alberswellness.com

Traci Callahan, LPC

Collaborative Counseling Consultation Resources

1480 Woodstone Dr., Suite 112

Saint Charles, Missouri 63304

(636) 451-7109

Bowel Issues for Children

Soiling Solutions – http://www.encopresis.com/

Varicose Veins

http://www.sheenveininstitutestl.com/

Mattress

American Freight Store

4525 Veterans Memorial Pkwy.

St. Peters, MO 63376

(636) 922-9555

Dr. Marvin's Orthopedic Chiropractic Mattress

Rx Plus Mattress

Nontoxic Mattresses:

Aviya

Avocado Mattress

Cariloha

Dream Clouod

Eco-Terra

Essentia

Hyphen Sleep

Layla Sleep

Live and Sleep Mattress

My Green Mattress

Nectar Sleep

Nest Bedding

Plush Beds

Purple Mattress

Puffy

Sweet ZZZ

Animal Chiropractor/ Physical Therapy/ Veterinary Services

Ava Frick, DVM, CVC, FAIS

105 E. 5th St.

Eureka, MO 63025

(636) 549-9100

www.animalfitnesscenter.com/

Diastasis Recti Rehabilitation

Motherhood Strong

Joselyn Miller, certified BIRTH FIT coach

(618) 979-7309

Tami Huber, certified Tupler Technique coach

(708) 466-7237

Pediatric Sleep Specialist

Nancy Birkenmeier

St. Luke's Sleep Medicine

(314) 205-6030

Functional Ultrasound and Advanced Imaging

Aaron Welk, DC, DACBR

Gateway Radiology

(636) 277-0014

Pediatric Endocrinology

Myrto Frangos, MD

Mercy Hospital

621 S. New Ballas Rd. #3002B

St. Louis, MO 63141

(314) 251-3002

Adult Endocrinology

Julie Silverstein, MD

Barns Jewish Hospital

660 S. Euclid Ave.

St. Louis, MO 63110

(314) 747-7300

Pediatric Neurologist

Denis Altman, MD

621 S. New Ballas Rd. #5009

St. Louis, MO 63141

(314) 251-5866

Pediatric Gastroenterologist

Elizabeth Utterson, MD

1 Children's Place

St. Louis, MO 63110

(314) 454-6173

(800) 678-4357

Adult Neurologist

DePaul Group

Seth Hepner, MD

Mike Synder, MD SSM (functional neurologist)

Matt Worth, DC, DACNB, FACFN (functional chiropractic neurologist)

Compounding Pharmacies

St. Charles – Powers Health Mart

Clayton – Jennifer's Pharmacy

Crestwood – Neels Pharmacy

Allergy and Immunology

Laura A. Esswein, MD

Pediatric Allergy and Immunology

10024 Watson Rd.

St. Louis, MO 63126

(314) 919-2500

Tongue and Lip-Tie Release

Little Flower Family Medicine (Laser)

207 E. Pitman St.

O'Fallon, MO 63366

(636) 875-1140

Cardinal Dental

Cyndi Blalock, DDS

cardinaldentist.com

(636) 441-7440

Mercy Birth Center – St. Louis

615 South New Ballas Rd.,
Ste. 1400

St. Louis, MO 63141

(314) 251-7955

Doctors Conoyer (father and two sons) Midwest EENT

4790 Executive Centre Pkwy.

St. Peters, MO 63376

(636) 441-3100

Maryanne Udy, DDS
(Oral surgeon at DePaul)

O'Fallon, MO

(636) 978-6967

(314) 291-3810

Medical Thermography

April Abbonizio

(314) 882-7529

Full body – $375

Half body – $275

1 region – $175

Whole 30 Coach

Kelly Warner

Showmewholeliving.com

showmewholeliving@gmail.com

(713) 839-5413

Fitness Trainers

Jessica White
(specializing in women over 50 years old)

Enact Wellness Solutions

1376 South 5th Street

St. Charles, MO 63301

(636) 410-4515

Emerge Fitness Training

Sefton Hale

920 Hemsath, Suite 100

St. Charles, MO 63303

(636) 757-3726

Brendan O'Neill

920 Hemsath, Suite 100

St. Charles, MO 63303

(636) 757-3726

APPENDIX B: RESOURCES

In this section, I provide the name and brief description of a wide range of products and services that can help you live in a way that promotes *Healing from Within*. These include references to professional health websites, as well as products and services relating to the air you breathe, the water you drink, and your home, yard, and personal care products.

Air

This section is one of the most foundational to good health. Clean air is an absolute must inside your home because we cannot necessarily control the outside air.

Rabbit Air MinusA2 – The MinusA2 offers an unmatched six-stage air-purification process that creates the cleanest, freshest air possible. https://www.rabbitair.com/pages/minusa2-air-purifier

Levoit Compact Air Purifier – This Levoit compact air-purifying device is a great buy for anyone who is looking for convenience. https://www.levoit.com/airpurifiers/

Honeywell HPA300 True HEPA Allergen Remover – If you weren't already aware of this fact, Honeywell is the No. 1 brand recommended by allergists. https://www.honeywellstore.com/

Winix PlasmaWave 5500-2 – This Winix air purifier is top-rated because it uses a patented PlasmaWave technology not found in other air cleaners. https://winixamerica.com/

AIRMEGA 300S Smart Enabled Air Purifier – This product ranks high on the list of best-rated air purifiers because it offers something not many other devices provide smart-enabled features. You can control every aspect of it from your iOS or Android device. https://www.cowaymega.com/airmega/

Hamilton Beach TrueAir Compact Pet Air Purifier – If you have pets and want an air purifier that can both freshen the air and remove pet hair, then look no further than this compact air purifier. At last count, it had more than 2,800+ reviews by consumers and continues to be one of the highest-rated air purifiers. This device uses a permanent HEPA-type filter that can be cleaned with a vacuum and doesn't need to be replaced, which saves a considerable amount of money. This is a solid investment for any pet owner. https://www.hamiltonbeach.com/trueair-compact

Winix WAC9500 Ultimate Pet True HEPA Air Cleaner – This is an excellent air purifier for pet owners, and you won't find any other product at this price that's as effective at removing all types of dust and allergens, including stubborn pet dander and hair. https://winixamerica.com/

Coway Mighty Air Purifier AP-1512HH – The Coway Mighty Air Purifier is excellent at not only removing dust and allergens but also reducing household odors, mold, and bacteria. It's the best-value air purifier you can get. https://www.cowaymega.com/

GermGuardian AC5000E 3-in-1 Air Cleaner – What makes this product so attractive is the fact that it uses a three-in-one air-cleaning system that tackles airborne pollutants of all types, making the room it's placed in a sterile, healthy environment. https://www.guardiantechnologies.com/

Alen Air BreatheSmart Customizable Air Purifier – If you're looking for a fully customizable air purifier that can also handle a very large space, this is it.

Alen Air Dehumidifiers – These are well-made dehumidifiers that will keep your air dry and less likely to grow mold and dust mites. https://www.alencorp.com

Breathing

Most of us take breathing for granted and fail to consciously use our breath to our greatest benefit. Below are some resources to help you master your breathing.

Nasopure – This device was developed by a local pediatrician to gently and easily clean your nasal passageways. Dr. Hana has decades of experience and is on a mission to educate people on the benefits of nasal washing. Her enthusiasm for patient empowerment and avoidance of medication overuse has become the core of her company, BeWell Health. The goal of her company is to help you feel better and breathe easier, naturally! We breathe 10,000 liters of air per day, and your nose is the first line of defense in a polluted world. Help avoid unnecessary illness and overmedication by washing your nose wash daily! https://www.nasopure.com/

Neti Pot – This device helps rinse mucous from your sinuses and allows for passage through your nose. The biggest difference between a Neti Pot and Nasopure is the method of irrigation. When using a Neti Pot, gravity works in your favor. Nasopure works by applying pressure to the bottle to force water up the nose. I personally find the Nasopure device to be much easier to use, and my two-year-old can use it as well. In addition, the Nasopure is much easier on your cervical spine, keeping your head and neck in a natural position.

Xlear Sinus Spray – This is a natural, effective, safe spray to use to break up mucous in your nasal passages so that it can be blown out easily. https://www.xlear.com

NeuralCranial Restructuring – This is a powerful technique used to correct a deviated septum and restore proper breathing. For a list of providers, go to https://ncrdoctors.com

Essential Oils – These are highly concentrated plant oils that help to nourish our physical and emotional well-being. There are many different companies and types of essential oils, so you must take precautions when choosing which oils to use. Make sure the oils are organic and ideally produced by steam distillation or fractional distillation, not via solvent extraction. Even the purest essential oils can be toxic, especially to children if used improperly, so keep them secured and out of reach to children. For additional information on essential oils, go to the National Associate for Holistic Aromatherapy. https://naha.org

Water

Drinking plenty of water each day isn't enough, unfortunately. If you want to have good health and longevity, your water must be clean and pure.

Berkey Water Filter – This is a quality water-filtration system that removes many compounds, including fluoride (you must choose that add-on). http://www.berkeyfilters.com

10 Stage Countertop Water Filter from New Wave Enviro – This is a great water filter that is very affordable. I used this filter before I started using my Berkey. It's great for traveling because of its size. https://www.newwaveenviro.com

Premium Shower Filter and Bath Filter from New Wave Enviro – This product can be installed on all your showerheads at home to filter out chlorine. The Splish Splash bath filter is also great and easy to use for bathing because we often soak for longer periods of time in the bathtub as opposed to the shower. This is especially important for infants and young children. https://www.newwaveenviro.com

Food

Instacart – This service delivers groceries from local stores in two hours. Choose from stores like Wholes Foods Market, Costco, and others. https://www.instacart.com

Thrive Market – Organic, healthy food is delivered to your door. https://www.thrivemarket.com

Health Professionals

Many organizations focus on natural health, but the ones listed below are the ones I have entrusted. The ones listed here also think holistically. Be mindful that although I trust each of these organizations, I do not know all the people on the directories.

Institute for Functional Medicine – This is one of the fastest-growing integrative medicine organizations in the world. www.functionalmedicine.org

International Chiropractic Pediatric Association (ICPA) – This is an organization dedicated to representing and training practitioners to provide evidence-informed care to the entire family, with a focus on pregnant mothers and children.

Medical Academy of Pediatric Needs (MAPS) – This is an outstanding organization for children with autism or chronic disease. http://www.medmaps.org

American Academy of Environmental Medicine and Naturopathic Academy of Environmental Medicine – These are health professionals who specialize in removing mold, industrial chemicals, or heavy metals and who are experts in understanding allergic and sensitive reactions to the environment. www.naturopathicenviroment.com www.aaemonline.org

DrBenLynch.com – This is a great resource for health professionals trained by Dr. Ben Lynch, who is the founder of Seeking Health, a company that helps educate both the public and health professionals on how to overcome genetic dysfunction through diet, lifestyle, and supplements.

Home, Lawn, and Garden

Our households, lawns, and gardens can be extremely toxic places, so what do you do? We try to avoid all chemicals in our home when possible. I recommend you eliminate them from your home too for exponential health benefits.

Weeds

Pitchfork – It's the best way to weed a bed.

Hula Hoe – This is the best type of hoe for fast removal of weeds.

Propane torch – Use this tool for open areas that need weeding (driveways and sidewalks).

Fertilizer and Soil Amendment

Hendrikus Organics – They are the leader in natural soil health and restoration. https://www.hendrikusorganics.com

Housecleaning

Norwex – They specialize in cleaning clothes that do not require chemicals or solvents to get them clean. https://norwex.com

E-Cloth – These are great cleaning cloths that do not require chemicals or solvents with which to clean. https://www.ecloth.com

Ecover – These are clean dishwashing tables. us.ecover.com

White Vinegar – Just dilute the white vinegar with water, and you are ready to clean. You can find it at any grocery store.

Laundry

On Guard Laundry Detergent by doTERRA is a great option. https://doterra.com

Thieves laundry soap by Young Living is another great option. https://youngliving.com

Molly's Suds is a great detergent that comes in scented or unscented. https://mollysuds.com

Wool dryer balls – Use them in place of smelly, wasteful antistatic dryer sheets. You can make your own too.

Personal Care Products

Cosmetics

Juice Beauty – I started using this line years ago when I made the decision to start using cleaner products. https://juicebeauty.com

Beauty Counter – These are clean, safe skin-care products. www.beautycounter.com

Crunchi – This is clean makeup that offers good choices for mascara, primer, foundation, and blush.

Dusty Girls – They offer good, clean options for bronzers, blushes, and BB cream, and they are all budget-friendly. http://dustygirls.com

GIA Minerals – They have great mascara and eyeshadow selections. https://www.giaminerals.com

Hynt Beauty – This is a great all-around clean makeup line. https://www.hyntbeauty.com

Vapour Organic Beauty – This is an amazing line; they have foundations, blushes, and lip products. www.vapourbeauty.com

Bath Products

Puracy Natural Baby Shampoo and Body Wash – This is a great option for infants and children. It's nontoxic and hypoallergenic. www.puracy.com

Kiss My Face – They offer natural skin-care products and soaps that smell amazing and are nontoxic. www.kissmyface.com

Deodorants

Rustic Maka Pachy – We have sold this in our office for years, and patients love it. It's one of my favorites. https://www.rusticmaka.com

Schmidt's – This is effective and budget-friendly. They have a sensitive formula available too. https://schmidtsnaturals.com

Ursa Major Hoppin' Fresh Deodorant – This is effective and comes in a unisex scent. https://www.ursamajorvt.com

Hair Products

Acure – These are budget-friendly shampoos, conditioners, and other styling products. They can be found at Whole Foods, your local health store, or https://www.acureorganics.com.

Flourish Organic Hair – This is a variety of hair-care products from shampoos and conditioners to styling products; they are also budget-friendly. www.flourishbodycare.com

Green & Gorgeous Dry Shampoo – This is available in both light and dark hair options. https://gandgorganics.com

Primally Pure Dry Shampoo – This is an amazing, nontoxic dry shampoo. https://primallypure.com

True Botanicals – These are ultra-luxe clean shampoo and conditioner in eco-friendly pump bottles. https://truebotanicals.com

Hand Creams

Birch Botanicals Spa is local to the St. Louis area and makes a variety of hand creams, body scrubs, facial serums, and lip balm. They are all clean, nontoxic and handmade. This is one of my favorite lines to support because of the amazing benefits of the products but also the commitment to purity and craft. www.birchbotanicalspa.com

100% Pure Hand Buttercream – This comes in a tube and leaves no greasy residue. https://www.100percentpure.com

Zoe Organics Everything Balm – This is great on hands or anywhere you need some extra hydration. https://www.zoeorganics.com

Skin-Care Products

Acure – These are budget-friendly body and facial skin-care products. https://www.acureorganics.com

AnnMarie – This skin-care line is so clean you could eat it! https://shop.annmariegianni.com

Dr. Bronner's – These are castile soaps for use as body washes. DYI cleaning recipes are also available. https://www.drbronner.com

Laurel Whole Plant Organics – This is a skin- care line based on herbs and flowers that is 100 percent raw, organic, and unrefined. https://www.laurelskin.com

Maya Chia Beauty – This is a superb antiaging line that uses chia-seed oil as the base for all formulations. https://mayachia.com

True Botanicals – This skin-care line has studies backing its potency and results. It's great for those who suffer from acne at any age, and it's also a great antiaging line. https://truebotanicals.com

Toothpastes

doTERRA On Guard toothpaste – This is what we use in our home, and we really love it. www.doterra.com

Jason's Toothpaste – This is clean, and fluoride-free options are available. http://www.jason-personalcare.com

Tom's of Maine Toothpaste – This is another clean, nontoxic formula. Fluoride-free options are available. http://www.tomsofmaine.com/home

Dental Herb Company Tooth & Gums Tonic – These are professional-strength mouthwashes and toothpastes made with pure essential oils and organic herbal extracts. www.dentalherb.com

Wellness Mama Blog – Here you can find great DYI recipes for toothpastes that will restore minerals back to your teeth. This is an approach some people have used to prevent cavities, along with a careful diet. http://wellnessmama.com

Sunscreens

Badger – This is one of the simplest, most natural sunscreens with minimal ingredients. www.badgerbalm.com

Babo Botanicals SPF 40 Daily Sheer Facial Sunscreens – These are sheer and lightweight. www.babobotanicals.com

Loving Naturals Adorable Baby Sunscreen SPF 30+ – These are great for babies and kids, made of simple ingredients. https://lovingnaturals.com

Raw Elements Sunscreen – This is the cleanest sunscreen made and it comes in a variety of formulas. https://rawelementsusa.com

Tracking Products for Exercise, Food, Heart-Rate Variability (HRV) and Sleep

When we can understand our body's patterns and behaviors in real time, it changes the way we see ourselves. It's also very useful to know exactly what and how much we're eating; it's even better when we can see what the food contains. The following tracking products can help you gather this important data as well as interpret it.

HRV4Training – This is a phone app that tracks your HRV via your cell-phone camera. http://www.hrv4training.com

CRON-O-Meter app – This app enables you to track what and how much you eat. It also shows in real time how much more you should eat for the day, broken down into protein, carbs, and fats. It also has settings for different diets, such as Paleo or Ketogenic. It's helpful when you want to lose or gain weight too. https://cronometer.com

Nutrient Optimiser – This ties in with the CRON-O-Meter to inform you what you should eat, what you shouldn't eat, and what you should eat more of. The goal is to get all your nutrients from food. This is a fantastic program designed by Marty Kendall. https://nutrientoptimiser.com

OURA ring – This is a pretty amazing gadget! I recently bought one for myself. This gadget tracks how well you're sleeping at night as well as your readiness to exercise (how hard you can exercise, or if you need to take it easy for the day based on HRV, heart rate, and body temp). orraring.com

Sleep Cycle app – This is a great starting app to measure the quality of your sleep. Although it gives you some insight, the OURA ring is more precise. https://www.sleepcycle.com

WISE. – What should I eat? Are you tired of people telling you what you can and can't eat? You can answer a few questions about what foods give you symptoms and about your health more generally and receive a report in minutes about what you can eat. You can expand your report into customized recipes prepared by a professional chef. Try it! www.drbenlynch.com

APPENDIX C: BOOK REFERENCES

What Is Health?

Jones, Rachel. "American Woman are still dying at alarming rates while giving birth." December 2018. (Accessed April 5, 2019.) https://www.nationalgeographic.com/culture/2018/12/maternal-mortality-usa-health-motherhood/

Martin, Nina. "U.S. Has the worst rates of maternal deaths in the developed world." May 2017. (Accessed May 5, 2018.) https://www.npr.org/2017/05/12/528098789/u-s-has-the-worst-rate-of-maternal-deaths-in-the-developed-world

The World FactBook. 2018. Infant Mortality Rates in U.S. https://www.cia.gov/library/publications/the-world-factbook/geos/us.html

Hamilton, B. E., J. A. Martin, M. J. K. Osterman, and S. C. Curtin. "Births: Preliminary data for 2013." National Vital Statistics Reports, 63(2). Hyattsville, MD: National Center for Health Statistics, 2014.

Res. 2014 Jun;7(3):295-304. doi: 10.1002/aur.1349. Epub 2013 Nov 18.

National Vaccine Information Center. https://www.nvic.org/downloads/49-doses-posterb.aspx

Van Cleave, Jeanne, Steven L. Gortmaker, and James M. Perrin. "Dynamics of Obesity and Chronic Health Conditions Among Children and Youth." Journal of the American Medical Association. Feb. 17, 2010. http://jama.jamanetwork.com/ article.aspx?articleid=185391

http://www.cdc.gov/ncbddd/developmentaldisabilities/features/birthdefects-dd-keyfindings.html.

http://www.cdc. gov/ncbddd/autism/facts.html

http://www.foodallergy.org/facts-and-stats

https://www.cdc.gov/ncbddd/developmentaldisabilities/features/birthdefects-dd-keyfindings.html

https://www.cancer.gov/types/childhood-cancers/child-adolescent-cancers-fact-sheet

What Is Chiropractic?

Meeker, WC, and S. Haldeman. “Chiropractic: a Profession at the Crossroads of Mainstream and Alternative Medicine.” Ann Intern Med 136, no. 3. 2002:216-227.

Hultman, C. “Autism May result from Intra-uterine Growth restriction, Foetal Distress.” Epidem 13. 2002:417-423.

Fallon, J, DC. Chiropractic and Pregnancy. New York: New Rochelle, 1998.

Henderson, I, MD. American Medical Association records released in 1987 during trial in US District Court Northern Illinois Eastern Division, No. 76C 3777. May 1987.

Towbin, A. “Latent Spinal Cord and Brain Stem Injury in Newborn Infants.” Dev Med Child Neurol 11. 1969:54-68.

The History of Chiropractic

Palmer, D.D. The Science, Art and Philosophy of Chiropractic. Portland, Oregon: Portland Printing House Company, 1910.

Leach, Robert. The Chiropractic Theories: A Textbook of Scientific Research. Lippincott: Williams and Wilkins, 2004. p. 15.

Ernst, E. “Chiropractic: a critical evaluation.” J Pain Symptom Manage 35, (no. 5). 2008: 544–62.

Keating, J. C. Jr., C. S. Cleveland III, and M. Menke. "Chiropractic history: a primer" (PDF). Association for the History of Chiropractic. Archived from the original (PDF) on Dec. 30, 2016. Retrieved June 16, 2008.

Lerner, Cyrus. Report on the history of chiropractic (unpublished manuscript, L. E. Lee papers, Palmer College Library Archives). "Archived copy" (PDF). Archived from the original (PDF) on Nov. 12, 2006. Retrieved Oct. 28, 2006.

Palmer, D. The Chiropractor. Press of Beacon Light Printing Co., 1914, p. 7.

Palmer D.D. D.D. Palmer's Religion of Chiropractic, 1911.

Chiropractic and Innate Intelligence

Hultgren, G. M., and J. S. Jeffers. "Shamanism, a religious paradigm: its intrusion into the practice of chiropractic." J Manipulative Physiol Ther 17, (no. 6). July-Aug.1994:404–410.

Donahue, J. H. D. D. "Palmer and the metaphysical movement in the 19th century." Chiropr Hist 7, (no. 1). July 1987:23–27.

Coulter, I. D. "The chiropractic paradigm." J Manipulative Physiol Ther 13, (no. 5). June 1990:279–287.

Keating, Joseph C., III, PhD. "Commentary: The Meanings of Innate." Archived April 30, 2013, at the Wayback Machine. J Can Chiropr Assoc 46, (no. 1). 2002.

Stephenson, R. W. Chiropractic Textbook. The Palmer School of Chiropractic. Davenport, IA, 1948.

Donahue, J. "Dis-ease in our principles. The case against innate intelligence." American Journal of Chiropractic Medicine 1, (no. 2). 1988:86.

Rothwell, D. M., S. J. Bondy, and J. I. Williams. "Chiropractic manipulation and stroke: A Population-based case-control study." Stroke 32. 2001:1054.

Pregnancy, Labor and Delivery with Chiropractic

Phillips, C. J., and J. J. Meyer. "Chiropractic care, including craniosacral therapy, during pregnancy: a static-group comparison of obstetric interventions during labor and delivery." J Manipulative Physiol Ther 18, (no. 8). 1995:525–529.

Fallon, J. M. Textbook on chiropractic & pregnancy. Arlington, VA: International Chiropractic Association, 1994: 52, 109.

DiMarco, D. B. "The female patient: enhancing and broadening the chiropractic encounter with pregnant and postpartum patients." J Am Chiropr Assoc 40, (no. 11). 2003:18–24.

Shaw, G. "When to adjust: chiropractic and pregnancy." J Am Chiropr Assoc 40, (no. 11). 2003:8–16.

Fallon J. M. "Chiropractic and pregnancy: a partnership for the future." ICA Int Rev Chiropr 46, (no. 6). 1990:39–42.

Vallone, S. "The role of chiropractic in pregnancy." ICA Int Rev Chiropr. 2002:47–51.

Krantz, C. K. "Chiropractic care in pregnancy." Midwifery Today 52. 1999:16–17.

What Is Functional Medicine?

Plotnikoff, G, and M. Barber. "Refractory depression, fatigue, irritable bowel syndrome, and chronic pain: A functional medicine case report." Perm J 20, (no. 4). Fall 2016:15–242. DOI: https://doi.org/10.7812/TPP/15-242.

Bland, J. "Systems biology, functional medicine, and folate." Altern Ther Health Med 14, (no. 3). 2008:18–20.

Jones, D. S., J. S. Bland, and S. Quinn. "What is functional medicine?" Textbook of Functional Medicine. Federal Way, WA: Institute for Functional Medicine, 2010. pp. 5–14.

Jones, D. S., and S. Quinn. Textbook of Functional Medicine. Gig Harbor, WA: Institute for Functional Medicine, 2010.

Jones, D, ed. Textbook of functional medicine. Gig Harbor, Wash: Institute of Functional Medicine, 2005.

Jones, D. S., L. Hofmann, and S. Quinn. 21st century medicine: A new model for medical education and practice. Gig Harbor, WA: The Institute for Functional Medicine, 2010, rev 2011.

Jones, D. S., and S. Quinn. Introduction to functional medicine. Gig Harbor, WA: The Institute for Functional Medicine, 2016.

The Wonderful Benefits of Intermittent Fasting

Seimon, R. V., J. A. Roekenes, J. Zibellini, et al. "Do intermittent diets provide physiological benefits over continuous diets for weight loss? A systematic review of clinical trials." Mol Cell Endocrinol 418. 2015:153–172.

Young, E. "Deprive yourself: The real benefits of fasting." New Scientist. Nov 12, 2012. (Accessed on December 8, 2016). https://www.newscientist.com/article/mg21628912-400-deprive-yourself-the-real-benefits-of-fasting/

Seimon, R. V., J. A. Roekenes, J. Zibellini, B. Zhu, A. A. Gibson, A. P. Hills, R. E. Wood, N. A. King, N. M. Byrne, and A. Sainsbury. "Do intermittent diets provide physiological benefits over continuous diets for weight loss? A systematic review of clinical trials." Mol. Cell Endocrinol 418. 2015:153–172. doi: 10.1016/j.mce.2015.09.014.

Barnosky, A. R., K. K. Hoddy, T. G. Unterman, and K. A. Varady. "Intermittent fasting vs daily calorie restriction for type 2 diabetes prevention: a review of human findings." Transl Res 164, (no. 4). 2014:302–11.

Varady, K. A. "Intermittent versus daily calorie restriction: which diet regimen is more effective for weight loss?" Obes Rev 12, (no. 7). 2011:E593–601. doi: 10.1111/j.1467-789X.2011.00873.x.

Harvie, M. N., M. Pegington, M. P. Mattson, J. Frystyk, B. Dillon, G. Evans, et al. "The effects of intermittent or continuous energy restriction on weight loss and metabolic disease risk markers: a randomized trial in young overweight women." Int J Obes 35, (no. 5). 2011:714–27.

Headland, M., P. M. Clifton, S. Carter, and J. B. Keogh. "Weight-loss outcomes: a systematic review and meta-analysis of intermittent energy restriction trials lasting a minimum of 6 months." Nutrients 8, (no. 6). 2016:E354.

Genetics vs. Epigenetics

Feinberg. "The Key Role of Epigenetics in Human Disease." N. Engl. J. Med 379, (no. 4). July 26, 2018:400-401.

Allis, C. D., and T. Jenuwein. "The molecular hallmarks of epigenetic control." Nat. Rev. Genet 17, (no. 8). Aug. 2016:487-500.

Berger, S. L., T. Kouzarides, R. Shiekhattar, and A. Shilatifard. "An operational definition of epigenetics." Genes and development 23, (no. 7). 2009:781–783.

Holliday, R. "Epigenetics: a historical overview." Epigenetics 1, (no. 2). 2006:76–80.

Nijhout, H. F. "Metaphors and the role of genes and development." Bioessays 12. 1990:441–6.

Sahotra, Sarkar. Genetics and Reductionism. Cambridge University Press. 1998. p. 140.

Staub, Jack E. Crossover: Concepts and Applications in Genetics, Evolution, and Breeding. 1994.

Weiling, F. "Historical study: Johann Gregor Mendel 1822–1884." American Journal of

Medical Genetics 40, (no. 1). 1991: 1–25, discussion 26.

The Link between Gluten and Your Health

Fasano, A., A. Sapone, V. Zevallos, and D. Schuppan. "Nonceliac gluten sensitivity." Gastroenterology 148. 2015:1195-204. 10.1053/j.gastro.2014.12.049

Jamnik, J., B. García-Bailo, C. H. Borchers, and A. El-Sohemy. "Gluten Intake is Positively Associated with Plasma α2-Macroglobulin in Young Adults." J Nutr 145. 2015:1256-62.

Eaton, W. W., L. Y. Chen, F. C. Dohan, Jr, D. L. Kelly, and N. Cascella. "Improvement in psychotic symptoms after a gluten-free diet in a boy with complex autoimmune illness." Am J Psychiatry 172. 2015:219-21.

Miller, D. "Maybe it's not the gluten." JAMA Intern Med 176. 2016:1717-8.

Estévez, V., J. Ayala, C. Vespa, and M. Araya. "The gluten-free basic food basket: a problem of availability, cost and nutritional composition." Eur J Clin Nutr 70. 2016:1215-7. 10.1038/ejcn.2016.139

Andrén Aronsson, C., H. S. Lee, S. Koletzko, et al. TEDDY Study Group. "Effects of gluten intake on risk of celiac disease: a case-control study on a Swedish birth cohort." Clin Gastroenterol Hepatol 14. 2016:403-409.e3. 10.1016/j.cgh.2015.09.030

The Gut-Brain Connection

Knight, R., and B. Buhler. Follow your gut: the enormous impact of tiny microbes. New York: Simon and Schuster, 2015.

Perlmutter, D. Brain maker: the power of gut microbes to heal and protect your brain - for life. London: Hachette, 2015.

Mayer, E. The mind-gut connection: how the hidden conversation within our bodies impact our mood, our choices and our overall health. New York: Harper Wave, 2018 [2016].

Hyland, N., and C. Stanton, eds. The gut-brain axis: dietary, probiotic and prebiotic interventions on the microbiota. Amsterdam: Academic Press; 2016.

Rhee, S. H., C. Pothoulakis, and E. A. Mayer. "Principles and clinical implications of the brain-gut-enteric microbiota axis." Nat Rev Gastroenterol Hepatol 6. 2009:306–314.

Mayer, E. A., T. Savidge, R. J. Shulman. "Brain-gut microbiome interactions and functional bowel disorders." Gastroenterology 146. 2014:1500–1512.

Foster, J. A., and K. A. McVey Neufeld. "Gut-brain axis: how the microbiome influences anxiety and depression." Trends Neurosci 36. 2013:305–312.

What Are Genetically Modified Organisms (GMOs)

Devos, Y., et al. "Ethics in the societal debate on genetically modified organisms: A (re)quest for sense and sensibility." Journal of Agricultural and Environmental Ethics 21. 2007:29–61. doi:10.1007/s10806-007-9057-6

Devlin, R., et al. "Extraordinary salmon growth." Nature 371. 1994:209–210.

Beyer, P., et al. "Golden rice: Introducing the β-carotene biosynthesis pathway into rice endosperm by genetic engineering to defeat vitamin A deficiency." Journal of Nutrition 132. 2002:506S–510S

Barta, A., et al. "The expression of a nopaline synthase-human growth hormone chimaeric gene in transformed tobacco and sunflower callus tissue." Plant Molecular Biology 6. 1986:347–357.

Takeda, S., and M. Matsuoka. "Genetic approaches to crop improvement: Responding to environmental and population changes." Nature Reviews Genetics 9. 2008:444–457. doi:10.1038/nrg2342

United States Department of Energy, Office of Biological and Environmental Research, Human Genome Program. Human Genome Project information: Genetically modified foods and organisms, (2007)

Controversy of the Germ Theory

"The History of the Germ Theory." The British Medical Journal. 1 (1415): 312. 1888.

Buchen, L. "The new germ theory." Nature. 2010. 468: 492-495.

Pasteur, Louis. "On the extension of the germ theory to the etiology of certain common diseases." Translated by H. C. Ernst. Comptes Rendus de l'Académie des Sciences. XC. May 1880:1033–44.

"Germ Theory." jrank.org. Archived from the original on January 31, 2016. Retrieved January 1, 2016.

Waller, J. Discovery of the Germ. London: Icon Books, 2004.

Worboys, M. Spreading Germs: Disease Theories and Medical Practice in Britain, 1865-1900. Cambridge: Cambridge University Press, new edition, 2008.

Gray, Nicholas F. Microbiology of Waterborne Diseases, 2nd ed., 2014.

Our Toxic Homes

Beyond Pesticides. The Safer Choice: How to Avoid Hazardous Home, Garden, Community and Food Use Pesticides. (Accessed Oct. 24, 2018.)

Centers for Disease Control and Prevention. Health Studies Branch: Understanding Chemical Exposures. (Accessed Oct. 24, 2018.)

Robey, W. C., III, and W. J. Meggs. Chapter 195. Pesticides. In: Tintinalli JE, Stapczynski J, Ma O, Cline DM, Cydulka RK, Meckler GD, T. eds. Tintinalli's Emergency Medicine: A Comprehensive Study Guide, 7e. New York: McGraw-Hill, 2011.

Fedoruk, M.J., R. Bronstein, and B. D. Kerger. "Ammonia exposure and hazards assessment for selected household cleaning product uses." J Expo Anal Environ Epidemiol 15. 2005:534–44.

Rosenman, K. D., M. J. Reilly, D. P. Schill, D. Valiante, J. Flattery, R. Harrison, et al. "Cleaning products and work-related asthma." J Occup Environ Med 45. 2003:556–63.

Quirce, S., and P. Barranco. "Cleaning agents and asthma." J Investig Allergol Clin Immunol 20, (no. 7). 2010:542–50.

Nazaroff, W. W., and C. J. Weschler. "Cleaning products and air fresheners: exposure to primary and secondary air pollutants." Atmos Environ 38, (no. 18). 2004:2841–65.

Singer, B.C., H. Destaillats, A. T. Hodgson, and W. W. Nazaroff. "Cleaning products and air fresheners: emissions and resulting concentrations of glycol ethers and terpenoids." Indoor Air 16, (no. 3). 2006:179–91.

Verdu, E. F., D. Armstrong, and J. A. Murray. "Between celiac disease and irritable bowel syndrome: The 'no man's land' of gluten sensitivity." Am. J. Gastroenterol 104. 2009:1587–1594. doi: 10.1038/ajg.2009.188.

Varady, K. A. "Intermittent versus daily calorie restriction: which diet regimen is more effective for weight loss?" Obes Rev 12, (no. 7). 2011:E593–601. doi: 10.1111/j.14767-789X.2011.00873.x.

Harvie, M. N., M. Pegington, M. P. Mattson, J. Frystyk, B. Dillon, G. Evans, et al. "The effects of intermittent or continuous energy restriction on weight loss and metabolic disease risk markers: a randomized trial in young overweight women." Int J Obes 35, (no. 5). 2011:714–27.

Headland, M., P. M. Clifton, S. Carter, and J. B. Keogh. "Weight-loss outcomes: a systematic review and meta-analysis of intermittent energy restriction trials lasting a minimum of 6 months." Nutrients 8, (no. 6). 2016:E354.

APPENDIX D: THE MOST TOXIC CLEANING PRODUCTS

To compile a list of the most toxic cleaning products, I turned to the experts at Good Guide, a leading authority on consumer-product assessment based on health, green-consciousness, and social responsibility. Each product was ranked based on its health rating, but ties were broken according to overall scores, which also include scores for societal and environmental impact.

Toxic chemicals in conventional household cleaners vary in their severity—from acute (immediate) hazards such as skin or respiratory issues, chemical burns, or watery eyes to chronic (long-term) hazards such as cancer, fertility issues, ADHD, compromised immune system, and more. Most toxic chemicals found in household cleaners fall into these categories:

- **Carcinogens** – cause or promote cancer
- **Endocrine disruptors** – mimic human hormones and cause false signals within the body, leading to issues such as infertility, premature puberty, miscarriage, menstrual issues, ADHD, and even cancer
- **Neurotoxins** – affect brain activity and can cause problems such as headaches and memory loss

Here are some home cleaning products considered to be the most toxic:

- **Corrosive drain cleaners, oven cleaners, and toilet-bowl cleaners:** These are the most acutely dangerous cleaning products on the market. The ingredients in these cleaners can cause severe burns to the skin and eyes, or if ingested, to the throat and esophagus.
- **Fabric softeners and dryer sheets:** The fragrances and other ingredients used to make them can cause asthma, allergies, or lung irritation.
- **Artificial fragrances:** The National Institute of Occupational Safety and Health has found that one-third of the substances used in the fragrance industry are toxic, yet because the formulas used for these fragrances are trade secrets, companies are not required to disclose the ingredients used.
- **Products that create suds (shampoo, liquid soap, bubble bath, laundry detergent):** Ingredients such as 1,4-dioxane, diethanolamine (DEA), triethanolamine (TEA), sodium laureth sulfate, PEG compounds, etc. are known carcinogens linked to organ toxicity.
- **Antibacterial products:** The ingredients used to kill bacteria in these soaps can encourage the development of drug-resistant superbugs.
- ***Chlorine bleach:*** Chlorine bleach is commonly used to treat drinking water, sanitize swimming pools, and whiten laundry, and it is a strong eye, skin, and respiratory irritant. Mixing chlorine bleach with other cleaners like ammonia can release dangerous chlorine gas. Exposure to chlorine gas can cause

coughing, shortness of breath, chest pain, nausea, or other symptoms.

- **Chlorine bleach and ammonia:** Separately these cleaners produce fumes with high acute toxicity to the eyes, nose, throat, and lungs and should not be used by people with asthma or lung issues. Used together, these products produce a toxic gas that can cause serious lung damage.

For additional information on chiropractic services, nutritional advice functional medicine or to discuss booking Dr. Felicity Keough for speaking engagements for your group or organization, feel free to email info@keoughchiropractic.com or visit her website at www.keoughchiropractic.com for more information.

ABOUT THE AUTHOR

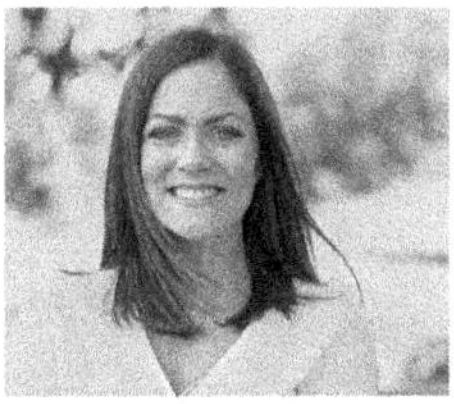

Dr. Felicity Keough-Bligh is a holistic family physician, proficient in manual medicine with her primary modality being chiropractic. She is most passionate about improving the health of women and children. She is an author, speaker, philanthropist and owner of one of the largest prenatal and pediatric chiropractic clinics in the Midwest. Dedicated to lifelong wellness, her mission is to serve, teach and inspire her patients so they can attain their full potential and sustain optimal health.

www.ingramcontent.com/pod-product-compliance
Lightning Source LLC
Chambersburg PA
CBHW070915030426
42336CB00014BA/2425
* 9 7 8 1 7 3 4 1 8 4 0 0 6 *